DIABETIC FOOT
A Clinical Atlas

DIABETIC FOOT
A Clinical Atlas

Sharad Pendsey
Diabetes Clinic and Research Centre
Dhantoli, Nagpur
India

With Forewords by

Marvin E Levin MD FACP
Professor of Medicine
Washington University School of Medicine
St Louis, Missouri, USA

Alethea VM Foster BA (Hons) PGCE DPodM MChs SRch
Lead Clinical Specialist Podiatrist
Diabetic Foot Clinic
King's College Hospital
London, UK

Michael E Edmonds MD FRCP
Consultant Physician
Diabetic Foot Clinic
King's College Hospital
London, UK

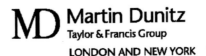
Martin Dunitz
Taylor & Francis Group
LONDON AND NEW YORK

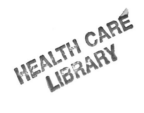

© 2003 Sharad Pendsey

First published in 2003
by Jaypee Brothers Medical Publishers (P) Ltd, EMCA House, 23/23B Ansari Road, Daryaganj, New Delhi 110 002, India

First published in the United Kingdom in 2004
by Martin Dunitz, an imprint of the Taylor & Francis Group plc, 11 New Fetter Lane, London EC4P 4EE. Exclusively distributed worldwide (excluding the Indian subcontinent) by Martin Dunitz, an imprint of the Taylor & Francis Group pic.

Tel.:   +44 (0) 20 7583 9855
Fax.:   +44 (0) 20 7842 2298
E-mail: info@dunitz.co.uk
Website: http://www.dunitz.co.uk

Although every effort has been made to ensure that all owners of copyright material have been acknowledged in this publication, we would be glad to acknowledge in subsequent reprints or editions any omissions brought to our attention.

Although every effort has been made to ensure that drug doses and other information are presented accurately in this publication, the ultimate responsibility rests with the prescribing physician. Neither the publishers nor the authors can be held responsible for errors or for any consequences arising from the use of information contained herein. For detailed prescribing information or instructions on the use of any product or procedure discussed herein, please consult the prescribing information or instructional material issued by the manufacturer.

A CIP record for this book is available from the British Library.

ISBN 1 84184 425 X

Distributed in the USA by
Fulfilment Center
Taylor & Francis
10650 Toebben Drive
Independence, KY 41051, USA
Toll Free Tel.: +1 800 634 7064
E-mail: taylorandfrancis@thomsonlearning.com

Distributed in Canada by
Taylor & Francis
74 Rolark Drive
Scarborough, Ontario M1R 4G2, Canada
Toll Free Tel.: +1 877 226 2237
E-mail: tal_fran@istar.ca

Distributed in the rest of the world by
Thomson Publishing Services
Cheriton House, North Way
Andover, Hampshire SP10 5BE, UK
Tel.:   +44 (0)1264 332424
E-mail: salesorder.tandf@thomsonpublishingservices.co.uk

Printed and bound by Gopsons Papers Ltd., Sector 60, Noida

Affectionately dedicated
to

Dr. Klein
Diabetes Klinik Bad Oeynhausen,
Germany,
my mentor who introduced me to
this interesting speciality of the Diabetic Foot

Dr Vinay Saoji
my close associate in footcare for the last two decades

Prof Sam GP Moses
Chennai, India who inspired me to compile
this Clinical Atlas on the Diabetic Foot

Foreword

Of the many complications affecting the person with diabetes, none is more devastating than those involving the foot. They include peripheral arterial disease, peripheral neuropathy, ulceration, infection and amputation. As the number of diabetics worldwide increases, we will see more and more diabetic foot problems. In the United States there are currently 17 million diabetics, and this number is increasing by some 800,000 per year.

Approximately 2 to 4% of the diabetic population will have a foot ulcer at any given time, and 15% will develop a foot ulcer during their lifetime. The escalating number of foot problems is due not only to the increasing diabetic population but to the fact that they are now living long enough to develop foot complications. Despite the many treatment modalities available today, the number of amputations, including toes to mid-thigh, is increasing. The Centers for Disease Control (CDC) noted that approximately one-third of persons with diabetes are at high risk for lower extremity amputation. The exact number of amputations due to diabetes in the United States is unknown. However, it is on the increase. In 1995, the number of amputations of toes to above the knee was 77,112; by 1996 it had risen to 85,530. I predict that by 2003 the number will be more than 100,000.

The diabetic foot and its problems, until recently, has been a neglected area of the diabetic's care. After all, foot problems are not very glamorous. Standard medical textbooks, until the late 1960s, included no more than one to two pages concerning the foot of the diabetic, and these pages were primarily devoted to foot hygiene. In those days surgeons frequently managed foot problems with amputation.

In the late 1960s Dr. Lawrence O'Neal and I realized that if you wanted to learn about the etiology and treatment of diabetic foot problems, you had to go to numerous textbooks. Therefore, in 1973 we published a textbook that we thought was the complete book on the treatment of the diabetic foot. It consisted of ten chapters, 262 pages. However, over the years the complexity of the diabetic foot and its treatment became apparent. In 2001 the sixth edition of **Levin and O'Neal's The Diabetic Foot** was published. It had grown to 38 chapters, 790 pages and included extensive information on basic pathophysiology. However, today what the primary care physician, internist, podiatrist (chiropodist), and nurse educator needs is a reference book that is primarily devoted to clinical matters, with case reports, illustrations and X-rays, depicting the various diabetic foot problems. Dr. Sharad Pendsey, an experienced clinician who sees and treats the problems of the diabetic foot on a day-to-day basis and is a world authority on the diabetic foot and its care has written it. Dr. Pendsey's **Diabetic Foot: A Clinical Atlas** is complete without being complicated. It quickly gets to the point of diagnosis and management. It includes case reports, which make it easy to understand a specific foot problem. The Atlas includes more than 600 color photographs and multiple X-rays.

I am acquainted with multiple diabetic foot books published over the last 30 years and I can truly say that this Atlas is outstanding. It should be required reading for every primary care physician and all medical personnel caring for the diabetic foot.

Dr. Pendsey is to be complimented for producing a clinical atlas that will educate the healthcare professional in the care of the diabetic foot and the prevention of amputation. Indeed, many persons with diabetes will owe Dr. Pendsey a debt of gratitude for helping to save their legs by educating their physicians in the appropriate care of the diabetic foot.

Marvin E Levin
MD FACP
Professor of Medicine
Washington University School of Medicine
St. Louis, Missouri, USA

Foreword

We were honoured to be asked to contribute a Foreword to this splendid diabetic foot book by our friend and colleague, Dr. Sharad Pendsey.

Dr. Pendsey is well-known throughout the world for his work in the field of diabetes, and for his charitable and humanitarian endeavors to improve outcomes for all people with diabetes in India. He is already the author of a respected volume on the management of diabetes, and we are glad that he has turned his attention to the diabetic foot. The foot is an area of the body which has often been referred to as "the poor relation", and many healthcare professionals show little interest in diabetic foot problems so we are delighted that Dr. Pendsey has come out on the side of the foot patient. Furthermore, the diabetic foot is frequently regarded with hopelessness, as if progression down the road to major amputation is inevitable once ulceration has developed, and in this book, Dr. Pendsey shows us ways of saving the diabetic foot in jeopardy.

Dr. Pendsey, in this lucid and attractive text, clarifies the ways in which diabetic foot problems can be prevented and treated successfully. This delightful book gives hope to the diabetic foot patient and support for those working in the field of diabetic foot care. It will provide enlightenment for the healthcare professional who is confronted with a diabetic foot in trouble. Progression down the road to amputation can often be prevented with the insights provided in this remarkable book.

This Clinical Atlas of the Diabetic Foot is a remarkably comprehensive volume, including over 600 photographs and over 50 case studies. There is something here for everyone: no matter how experience we think we are we can learn from Dr. Pendsey's wisdom, gained from many years of practical experience managing diabetic feet. Some of his material is particularly relevant to problems seen in India, such as rat bite, and lateral malleolar bursitis in people who sit cross legged: other problems are found wherever in the world there are people with diabetes and diabetic feet. Dr. Pendsey gives practical solutions to these problems.

An area of key importance in diabetic foot care is that of prevention, and Dr. Pendsey emphasises the need for preventive footcare and footwear, regular inspections, and working as a team. The patient and his family are important members of the team. Any person with diabetes and foot complications will have a life-long need for help with the feet. The burden of the diabetic foot is very great, but Dr. Pendsey's superb volume will help all practitioners to improve outcomes for the diabetic foot.

Alethea VM Foster
BA(Hons) PGCE DPodM MChS SRCh
Lead Clinical Specialist Podiatrist
Diabetic Foot Clinic
King's College Hospital
London, UK

Michael E Edmonds
MD FRCP
Consultant Physician
Diabetic Foot Clinic
King's College Hospital
London, UK

Preface

The diabetic foot is a quiet dread of disability, long stretches of hospitalization, mounting impossible expenses, with the ever dangling end result of an amputated limb. Health providers concerned with the care of diabetic patients are aware of the immense burden of misery that can be inflicted by the diabetic foot. Eventhough it affects only a proportion of diabetic patients, understanding the causes of this catastrophe, identifying the sufferers and those at high risk and developing effective preventive strategies and remedies for its consequences has rightly become a major preoccupation for diabetologists in recent years.

This clinical atlas of the diabetic foot, I suppose, should be ample testimony to the dedicated hardship put in by our footcare team in the last two decades. Frankly, building a comprehensive text was never conjured, and the endeavour focussed purely on offering a practical reference Atlas. I so much hope this effort comes useful to those involved in diabetic foot management.

This atlas is primarily devoted to clinical matters with illustrations and case reports depicting the varied diabetic foot problems. It has been divided into eight sections and forty-eight chapters with fifty-three case studies and six hundred forty clinical photographs. The bibliography cites excellent works, to quest more detailed texts.

In the last twenty years of my practice in India, my abiding impression has been that only a few persons with type 1 diabetes have diabetic foot complications. This is not only because of its low prevalence among Indians but also that sadly very few children with type 1 diabetes thirty years back, have managed to survive to become a victim of the long-term consequences of diabetes such as the diabetic foot. It has been observed that extrinsic factors operate predominantly in our patients in inflicting diabetic foot lesions because of the practice of walking barefoot, use of improper footwear, and the lack of awareness, among the patients and the primary care physicians, about the deadly consequences of trivial foot lesions in diabetics. The intrinsic factors like gross foot deformities, Charcot foot, plantar ulcers, and the peripheral vascular disease are less common for the same reasons, younger age and shorter duration of diabetes. Among approximately 40,000 leg amputations performed yearly on Indians, the vast majority are probably preventable as the amputation is invariably for an infected neuropathic foot.

It is easy to be optimistic that in years to come, with better understanding of the management of diabetes, the longevity of our diabetic patients would increase. But tempering this optimism is the realisation that this would throw up a huge number of longstanding diabetics, and therefore its complications, imposing a severe strain on the already hobbling health services.

In India, the concept of "team approach" is only now starting to pickup. Specialities like podiatry and orthoses are yet to be developed. Physicians often cannot be brought to even unwrapping foot dressings and then more often than not making a blind surgical referral. I shall be thrilled if this atlas encourages the physician to developing diabetic foot services at their centres, with a team geared to 'save' and not 'amputate'.

I am pleased that profits from the sale proceeds of this atlas will go towards furthering the services of "DREAM Trust", a registered charity (www.dreamtrust.org) with two overriding objectives, prevention of the diabetic foot and providing free insulin to children of the poorest of poor.

Sharad Pendsey

Acknowledgements

Not unsurprisingly, compiling this Atlas has proved to be a mammoth task which could hardly have been possible without the effusive help of so many, some indirect and some even unknowing. How did one ever seriously managed to thank those many and on a single page? Dreading the inevitable 'missing names', I at one point considered even skipping this page altogether.

First of all, the inordinate contribution of Rutuja Sharma, who spent countless hours, over these many weeks running into months, in tabulating the data, matching the photographs and getting them scanned and much more. Without her untiring zeal, this atlas would have been one more of 'conceived but unborn'.

My friends overseas Mukund Vaidya, Consultant Radiologist, Dewsbury UK; Ash Pawade, Consultant in Cardiovascular Surgery, Bristol, Vivien Lees, Consultant in Plastic Surgery, Manchester, UK, went through the manuscript with that hawk-eye coming up with invaluable suggestions and deserve a special mention, but then how did one thank friends? I am particularly indebted to Paul Brand, and Marvin Levin, USA, the two legendary figures in the speciality of the diabetic foot, former for contributing a page on thermal changes in the foot and latter for writing the foreword for this atlas. I am grateful to Mike Edmonds and Ali Foster, London, UK for writing the foreword for this atlas and to Karel Bakker, Netherlands, for permitting me to reproduce some of the photographs in this atlas. They have my profuse thanks for constantly egging me on through the paces of this endeavor.

I have no words to express my gratitude to our footcare team of Vinay Saoji, Consultant in Plastic Surgery, Abhay Nafdey, Rutuja, Smita, Chanda, Rita, Suresh, and members of allied specialities P.K. Deshpande and Ajay Patil both cardiovascular surgeons, Shrikant Kothekar interventional radiologist, Amit Deshmukh, radiologist, H.J. Sangtani and Satish Kale, orthopedic surgeons, A.M. Joglekar and Vikram Marwah, surgeons and Shimmi Dubey, orthotist.

Manjusha Joshi and Yogesh Wandhare for the arduous office assistance and typing of the manuscript, my daughter Gunjan for her drawing skills and Shakti Offset for scanning the photographs, are among the many obligations that often spring to mind.

My family, and not just wife Swati, children Gunjan and Sanket were always there with their wholehearted support, easily forgiving me when the Atlas, too often, stole 'my hours with them'. My parents 'Nana' and 'Aai' have always been the epitome of inspiration and encouragement, blessings that makes everything possible. Finally, and of course, it is thousands of my patients, providing the clinical material and taking me into the intricacies of the diabetes foot problems, who gave me a new insight beyond the conventional textbook wisdom. They will always have my gratitude.

Contents

SECTION THREE: NAIL AND SKIN LESIONS

SECTION FOUR: INFECTED NEUROPATHIC FOOT

SECTION FIVE: NEUROISCHEMIC FOOT

SECTION SIX: AMPUTATION

SECTION SEVEN: PREVENTION OF THE DIABETIC FOOT

SECTION EIGHT: OTHER ASPECTS

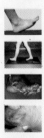

1 Introduction

Triple jeopardy Neuropathy, Ischemia, Infection

The diabetic foot is often an inching painless surprise that holds in its dark portals a soon rising flood of complications. It is a quiet dread of disability, long stretches of hospitalization, mounting impossible expenses, with the ever dangling end result of an amputated limb. The phantom limb plays its own cruel joke on the already demoralized psyche. The diabetic foot no wonder, is one of the most feared complications of diabetes.

Among people with diabetes, 15% will experience a foot ulcer in their life time. It is now appreciated that 15-20% of patients with such foot ulcers go on to need an amputation. Similarly, 85% of major lower limb amputations are preceeded by a foot ulcer. Diabetic foot problems are a major cause of hospitalization and prolonged hospital stay. Foot lesions in a person with diabetes is indeed an expensive proposal. The cost of treatment varies between countries. The approximate cost of healing of a foot ulcer without amputation is US $ 5000–10,000. With amputation this cost rises to US $ 10,000–40,000. In India the cost incurred for primary healing of foot ulcer without amputation is US $ 200-1000, while for amputation it is US $ 1000-2000. Although, the cost of treatment seems to be much lower, majority of our patients are not medically insured and find this cost exorbitant. Despite the targeted treatment aimed at preventing amputation, the incidence of lower limb amputation in persons with diabetes has continued to rise globally.

The diabetic foot is characterized by a classical triad of neuropathy, ischemia, and infection. (Fig. 1.1). The presence of infection and altered host response because of chronic hyperglycemia rapidly worsens the clinical picture from what appeared trivial just the other day, to one that now is suddenly limb or even life threatening.

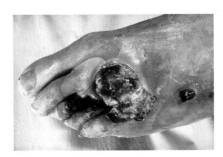

Fig. 1.1: Triad of neuropathy, ischemia and infection

Diabetic foot is seldom seen in isolation; it usually accompanies other macro and microvascular complications of diabetes. It is hence essential to pay due attention to the other systems, renal and cardiovascular in particular, while managing the diabetic foot. Advanced diabetic foot is like a **prothrombotic state** and it is not uncommon to see a fresh cardiovascular or cerebrovascular event, while managing the diabetic foot.

Quantitative plantar pressure measurements have remarkably changed the understanding of the pathogenesis of foot ulcer. It has also refined the footwear prescription, which is so essential for high risk feet. Newer antibiotics, recent therapies, and better dressing materials, have improved the clinical course of diabetic foot lesions to some extent. Inconceivably and equally painfully, it is the ignorance, whether on part of the patient or the primary care physician, that has remained the stumbling block in improving the outcome of diabetic foot lesions. Diabetics need to be managed under the care of a multidisciplinary team with expertise in the many facets of care. In some centres in the developed world it has been possible to reduce the amputation rate by 50%. The specific innovations of education, prescribing appropriate footwear, multdisciplinary team approach, and the increasing use of infra-popliteal bypass by the vascular surgeons have been the major factors responsible for these improvements. The message concerning the team approach needs to be heard around the world.

Why Feet and not Hands ?

Why should both peripheral vascular disease and peripheral neuropathy in persons with diabetes mellitus be restricted to lower limbs only and spare the upper limbs? The answer to this question has always eluded us. Darwin's theory of evolution states that, human beings have evolved from their ancestors, apes (Fig. 1.2). Assumption of erect posture on hind legs has caused profound anatomical and structural changes to the inferior extremity. Evolutionary structural changes that take place are by and large beneficial. Two changes are particularly noticeable in the lower limbs, one is comparative lengthening of the lower extremity, and the other is the rotation (internal) to render the foot planti-grade. Although, these changes have made it possible for the human beings to adopt an erect posture thus distinguishing them from rest of the animal kingdom, for persons with diabetes, it has been slightly disadvantageous. The weight bearing got restricted to two instead of four limbs. Our ability to see our plantars decreased significantly and the great toe went farthest away from the body thus requiring longest nerves and arteries.

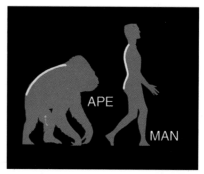

Fig. 1.2: Evolution from ape to man

Both neuropathy and vascular disease are to some extent length related. The superior extremity has evolved to perform multiple dexterous functions, whereas the planti-grade foot has evolved primarily to facilitate weight bearing and locomotion. The interossei and lumbricals which make the hand an efficient organ improving the mobility of the digits are comparatively inefficient in the foot. Despite all the disadvantages, the human foot which consists of 26 bones, 29 joints, and 42 muscles remains a mechanical marvel. In a lifetime it is estimated that, a human being walks about 100,000 miles (1,50,000 KM), equalling to almost four times around the world. Historically, the human race is plagued by that incredible and inexplicable stupidity in not waking up to what is critical and theirs to care. The taken for granted foot has since long joined the queue of 'missed only when lost'.

2 Gait (Walking) Cycle

Learning to Walk is Child's Play
Learning how We Walk, is not

We have been blessed with a pair of lower limbs which work in excellent co-ordination. All the muscles, joints, afferent, and efferent nerve impulses work so efficiently and are so well co-ordinated that we hardly realize how we stand, walk, run, dance, jump, climb effortlessly and with fluid ease. We all use the same walking tools and mechanics, yet it is so easy to spot a friend even from a distance from that trademark walk. It is interesting to watch people walking on the street, young or old, tall or dwarf, male or female, obese or lean as each one of them seems to have grown a unique walking style. And, to crown it all, some have fashion designed the walk into a catching, rhythmic art form (cat walk). Here are some relevant walking tit-bits.

- The stride lengths are symmetrical, measure about 76 - 81 cm. (30 - 32 in).
- The average number of steps are approximately 100/min.
- The average speed of walking is 4 km/h (2.5 mph)
- The net energy cost of walking is 2.5 cal/min.
- The higher the speed, the more the energy cost
- Normal gait is extremely efficient and any alteration decreases efficiency increasing the energy consumption.
- Walking on a deformed foot decreases efficiency and increases energy consumption.
- Above knee amputees require double the energy to walk than normal subjects.

While trying to understand the walking cycle we need to learn certain basic terminologies and phases. Walking is a well co-ordinated interaction of forces and movements of all the major joints of lower limb and is more than merely placing one foot ahead of the other. While walking, all the body segments are in motion and can be accurately described. To explain the analogy with an aeroplane, it has a landing phase (on touching the ground), a stationary phase (when it is on the ground), a take off phase (off the ground) and a flying phase (in the sky). Similarly, gait cycle has a landing phase when the foot strikes the ground (heel strike), midstance phase (when the foot is in complete contact with the ground) and take off phase (toe off) when the foot leaves the ground and swing phase when the foot is in the air. The only difference is that, an aeroplane takes off and lands on its rear wheels, whereas the foot takes off on forefoot and lands on the hindfoot.

A complete gait cycle has a stance phase (ground contact Fig. 2.1-2.4) and swing phase (in the air Figs 2.5 to 2.8).

Stance Phase

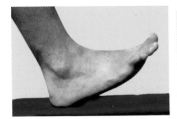
Fig. 2.1: Heel strike

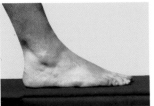
Fig. 2.2: Mid stance

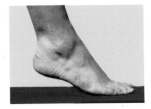
Fig. 2.3: Heel off

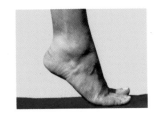
Fig. 2.4: Toe off

Swing Phase

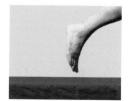

Fig. 2.5: Acceleration
(left the ground)

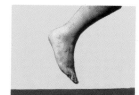

Fig. 2.6: Mid stance
(in the air)

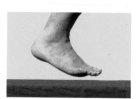

Fig. 2.7: Mid swing
(in the air)

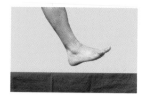

Fig. 2.8: Deceleration
(about to land)

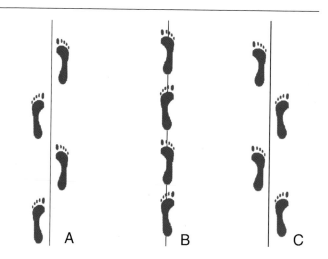

Figs 2.9A to C: **(A)** Normal walk, **(B)** Models walk, **(C)** Overdone models walk, * Personal communication with Ms Anna Uhlich, Vienna, an international model.

One complete gait cycle is the period between two successive heel strikes by the same foot. During normal walking, the swing phase of one leg coincides with the stance phase of the other leg. However, there is a period during which both feet are on the ground (double support time). The double support period of the gait cycle disappears when the subject starts to run. In normal walking cycle, each leg is in stance phase for about 60% and in swing phase for about 40%. Normally, we do not walk in a straight line, there is a small deviation of about 2 inches (5 cms) on either side of the line (Fig. 2.9 A). The greater the deviation, the lesser is the efficiency and the more is the energy expenditure. Fashion models walk in a different rhythm (Fig. 2.9 B, C). They walk on the straight line or some even cross the midline alternately. This deviation from a normal walk requires more bodily movements and pelvic rotation, thus making the models walk pleasing to the eyes.

Mechanism of Running

The major difference while running is that the gait cycle is altered considerably. The amount of force generated is increased so also is the range of motion of the lower limb joints. During walking one foot is always on the ground and as the speed increases, in running, the float phase is incorporated during which both feet are off the ground. There is no longer a period of double limb support. As the running speed increases, the time the foot spends on the ground is decreased considerably.

The overall gait pattern of the neuropathic diabetic is tentative as a result of feeling unsafe during standing and walking. This conservative walking style is characteristically the product of poor proprioception, diminished sensory information, and an overall lack of stability resulting in reduction in velocity and stride length with altered displacement of forces.

The technical information in this chapter is adopted from Roger A. Mann. Biomechanics of the Foot and Ankle. In Roger A. Mann, Michael J. Coughlin, eds. Surgery of the Foot and Ankle. Mosby-Year Book Inc: 1993: 3-43.

3 Biomechanics

*The whole problem of neuropathic feet is really
one of mechanics, not of medicine*

— Paul Brand

The majority of foot ulcers in diabetics are a consequence of mechanical trauma unnoticed by the patient due to neuropathy. Commonest sites of ulcerations are in the forefoot. Ulcers occur at sites of high pressure on either plantar or dorsal surfaces and are caused by bony prominences, ill fitting footwear, and toe deformities.

Normal Weight Bearing

The weight of the body, during walking , is borne mostly by one leg at a time. The tibia transmits weight to the talus and to the rest of the foot. When the foot first touches the ground while walking, the heel bone (calcaneus) takes all the weight, however, the other foot as well, is still sharing some of the body weight. As soon as the heel is firmly on the ground the other foot leaves the ground. The forefoot then comes down on to the ground but usually the lateral border of the foot takes on the weight first, transmitting it through the cuboid bone and base of the 5th metatarsal. A moment later the whole foot is on the ground (stance phase) (Fig. 3.1, 3.2). Thus the weight is transmitted from calcaneus, cuboid, base of the 5th metatarsal, and the heads of all five metatarsals. As the other foot swings forward the heel begins to leave the ground and the whole weight is on the forefoot (Fig. 3.3). Finally a strong contraction of the toes pushes the body forward to transfer its weight on the other foot, which by now is in position. In one walking cycle, when the foot comes down, it rests on the back of the heel, then additionally on the underside of the metatarsals and finally on to the heads of metatarsals to push off for the next step.

While the foot is standing on the ground, it is rather like an arch sparing the midfoot from weight bearing (Fig. 3.4). The medial arch of the foot is formed by calcaneus posteriorly and first three metatarsals anteriorly. The lateral two metatarsals form the lateral arch, which is relatively flat and works like a tie-beam to support the medial arch. The plantar aponeurosis connects the arches anteroposteriorly and is like a bow string. When it contracts the arch rises and when it relaxes, the arch flattens (Fig. 3.5).

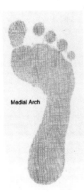

Fig. 3.1: Foot print showing normal weight bearing in stance phase, note medial arch

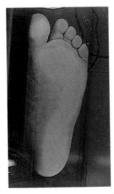

Fig. 3.2: Barograph showing normal weight bearing in stance phase

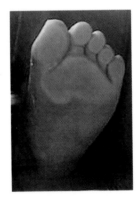

Fig. 3.3: Barograph showing forefoot bearing the weight in heel off phase

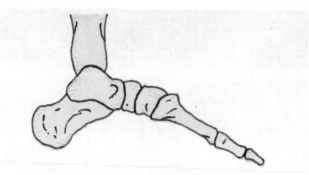

Fig. 3.4: Longitudinal medial arch of the foot

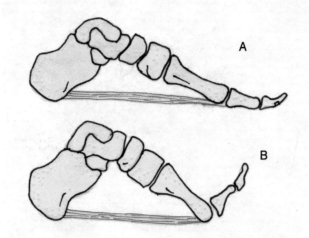

Fig. 3.5: **A** arch flat, **B** contraction of plantar aponeurosis resulting in elevation of the arch.

The intricate mechanism, involving joints of the foot, ligaments, muscles, bones, and the supple and resilient plantar tissue, makes our walking and running so comfortable that even barefoot walking does not lead to any foot problems. It is fascinating to watch the slow motion television clips of footballers and cricket pace bowlers. Their feet display several motions like acceleration, deceleration, sudden stop, jumping, twisting, and turning and so on and all this fleeting past within that one stare. The supreme co-ordination owes itself to protective sensations (afferent and efferent impulses), joint sense, continuous weight transfer and silver quick reflexes.

Weight bearing in Diabetic Neuropathy

Chronic hyperglycemia and polyneuropathy causing damage to sensory, motor, and autonomic nerve fibers lead to certain functional and structural changes in the foot. Chronic hyperglycemia leads to nonenzy-matic glycosylation of proteins causing limited joint mobility, reduction in the elastic tissues of plantar skin, and underlying collagen tissue. Foot deformities occur as a result of atrophy of intrinsic muscles of the foot and previous scars and toe amputations alter the architecture of the foot. Loss of elasticity, resilience, flexibility, and free joint movements lead to a relatively rigid and unstable foot with altered weight-bearing areas. Bony prominences develop underneath the foot pushing the fibrofatty shock-absorbing tissue forward, exposing the condyles of the metatarsal heads. The combination of various risk factors in the presence of neuropathy increase the plantar pressures significantly in the forefoot and hallux and increases the risk of foot ulceration (Fig. 3.6).

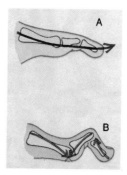

Figs 3.6A and B: **(A)** Normal escape of force from body weight, **(B)** Counter force on the metatarsal heads due to deformities

Plantar Pressure Measurement

Semi quantitative estimation of plantar pressures can be carried out using the ink pad, on which the patient's foot leaves an impression in different shades. Although, this method is quite specific, it is not very sensitive (Fig. 3.7).

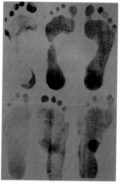

Fig. 3.7: Foot prints in different clinical situations, right upper being normal

Quantitative measurement of plantar pressures is now possible with many devices commercially available, and all require the use of a computer and special software (Figs 3.8 - 3.11).

For barefoot measurement, the patient walks onto the platform. In this situation, information from a single foot contact is collected. For in-shoe measurement the matrix of transducers is manufactured into a thin pliable "insole", which is placed in the shoe in direct contact with the foot. In this case, information from multiple steps can be obtained.

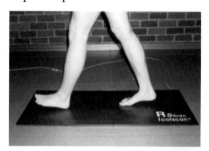

Fig. 3.8: * Barefoot plantar pressure measurement

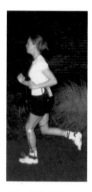 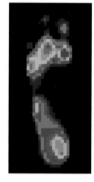

Fig. 3.9: * In-shoe plantar pressure measurement, note sensor in the left shoe

Fig. 3.10: * Scan of high-risk foot showing increased plantar pressure under the metatarsal heads

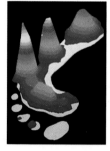

Fig. 3.11: * 3D scan showing increased plantar pressure at 5th metatarsal head

*Pictures with permission of RS scan International, Belgium

HOW DOES FOOT INJURY OCCUR ?

Healthy individuals remain ulcer free not necessarily because they have low plantar pressures, but because they can feel pain. Studies carried out to measure peak plantar pressures in normal individuals reveal that peak pressure ranges between 50 Kilo pascals (KPa) to 300 KPa with the lowest measures being on the midfoot region and the highest pressures being on the heel, and on the heads of the 1st three metatarsals and hallux. Various studies in patients with diabetic neuropathy have revealed that peak plantar pressures are increased two to three folds. However, there is no agreement to suggest the threshold pressure for injury. The barefoot plantar pressure can only predict the degree of risk, the ulceration occurs because of the combined effect of various factors. There will always be patients who ulcerate even at relatively low pressures because of significant activity level, walking barefoot or walking with poor footwear. Conversely, there will be patients who, because of low activity or protective footwear will not ulcerate even with very high barefoot plantar pressure.

Elevated plantar pressure is now accepted as a major factor in the pathogenesis of plantar ulcers in diabetics. Plantar pressure measurement can identify areas of high pressure unsuspected on clinical examinations and in shoe measurement can refine the process of footwear prescription by defining the exact degree of pressure relief at high-risk areas.

Continuous Pressure Causing Tissue Ischemia

It has been realized that some regions of the plantar tissue become ischemic when the foot is loaded. Everytime the foot is lifted from the ground, the pressure is released and capillaries reopen restoring the blood supply (Fig. 3.12). When a normal person

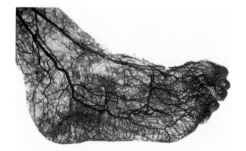

Fig. 3.12: Capillary network in the foot (from Amputation? Nein danke! Verlag Neuer Merkur GmbH, 1999)

stands for sometime, he feels uncomfortable and hence changes the position of the feet, thus restoring the blood supply. When a person with diabetic neuropathy stands still for some time, the capillaries get occluded, but this does not give him discomfort due to lack of sensations. He continues to stand in the same position causing tissue ischemia resulting in tissue injury. Recovery from this ischemia may also be affected in diabetics because of altered hemorrheology and microcirculation.

Thrust

When the foot strikes the ground, there are equal forces experienced by both the foot and the floor. The link between force and pressure is determined by area of force application. The smaller the surface area the greater is the pressure. In diabetic neuropathy, weight bearing areas are altered and foot deformities and bony prominences are common. Much more damage can be done by a force transmitted through a few plantar prominences than by the same force distributed over a larger area of plantar surface. A bony projection or callus projecting downwards from the foot has much the same effect as a piece of the ground projecting upwards into the foot. Thus a protruding metatarsal head has the same effect as that of a person walking with a pebble inside the shoe.

Dorsiflexion at the first MTP joint is essential during the toe off phase of gait. When the ability to dorsiflex is limited (Hallux rigidus), a very high pressure develops under the hallux explaining the high prevalence of ulcers on the ball of the great toe (Fig. 3.13). Deformities are considered to be a surrogate marker for elevated plantar pressure. In addition, soft

tissue "metatarsal cushions" are displaced distally, leaving the condyles of the metatarsal heads exposed.

The total weight bearing area of the foot is reduced significantly, increasing the pressure on the limited weight-bearing surface. The presence of scar from a previous ulcer is a leading risk factor for future ulceration (Fig. 3.14). The previously ulcerated foot is never quite the same again. A certain section of the soft, springy tissue of the sole is replaced by a piece of hard and non elastic scar tissue. The skin over the scar is thin and tears easily. Even minor amputation of the forefoot is associated with significant elevated pressure in other neighboring areas as compared to the contralateral intact foot. Plantar callus is common at the elevated pressure sites. Excessive growth of the callus acts to elevate the pressure further. Removal of callus reduces the plantar pressure by 30%, emphasizing the importance of callus care in the patient at risk for neuropathic ulceration.

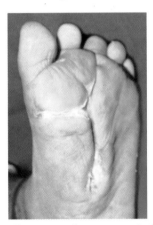

Fig. 3.14: Scar over plantar aspect of the foot, a risk factor for ulceration

Shear Stress

Apart from thrust (vertical pressure), there are forces during gait which are called shear forces, that tend to make the foot slip from its relatively fixed position on the ground. In a normal foot resting on the ground, it is quite possible to move the foot backwards and forwards on the ground without the skin actively moving on the ground. There is sufficient elasticity in the sole of the foot. Shear is a horizontal force which is most marked when a person is walking fast, during acceleration, deceleration or with a sudden stop after running. The horizontal movement between the skin below and the bone above is altered in a previously

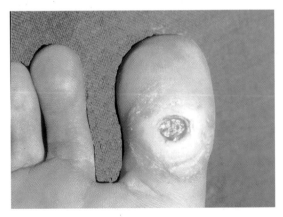

Fig. 3.13: Ulcer on ball of the great toe

ulcerated foot. The scar tissue is relatively fixed and does not move horizontally on the bone above it. However, little is known at present, about the magnitude and direction of shear stress during everyday activities or its role in causing plantar injury.

Thermal Changes in The Feet
(This Paragraph is Entirely Based on the Experiments Carried out by Dr. Paul Brand, Seattle, USA and his Personal Communication)

Two photographs (Fig. 3.15, 3.16) are thermographs of the soles of the feet of a healthy individual which were taken at rest periods during an eight mile run. The temperature scale of the thermograph covers ten degrees celsius from blue at the cool end to white at the warm end. These pictures demonstrate the way in which a normal foot when subjected to repetitive stress gradually becomes inflamed and therefore hotter. As the inflammation develops, so the temperature rises and also commencing pain at the area of highest stress results in some limping. The person with normal sensation adopts by changing the posture of the foot,

so that if the medial side of the foot has taken more stress early in the day, the lateral side takes its turn, thus allowing shift the stress and inflammation. In an insensitive foot the inflammation begins to take place, but there is no pain, and thus the inflammation increases until finally the tissues break down and ulcerate.

Thus a normal foot is saved from ulceration by the perception of the early pain of inflammation. The best way to save an insentitive foot from ulceration is to find a way for the patient to recognize progressive inflammation even without pain, before it reaches the stage of tissue breakdown and ulceration. Our experimentation has demonstrated that in insensitive feet, every stage of inflammation is accompanied by progressive rise of temperature which is limited to the area of inflammation. Most insensitive feet have a patch of increased temperature where there has been most stress. If these temperatures are recorded by a skin thermometer at home every evening it becomes easy for the patient to monitor his or her progress, and walk less on the day after the temperature has shown a rise. The temperature should be taken of a

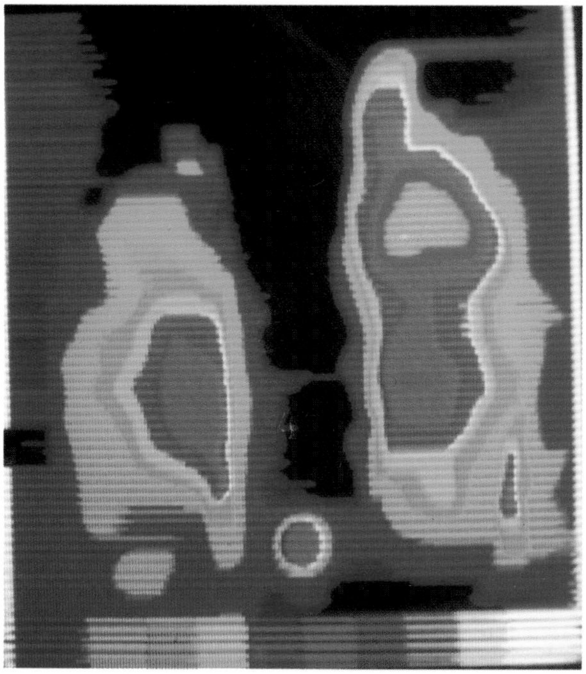

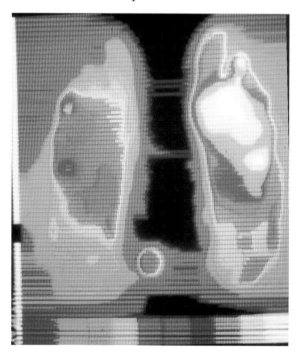

Fig. 3.15: * Thermograph taken during a rest after two miles of running. In right foot, medial side of sole is warmest, 1st metatarsal head area is hottest, great toe is the only warm toe.

Fig. 3.16: * Thermograph taken during a rest after eight miles of running. In right foot, hottest spots are second toe, metatarsal heads of 2nd to 4th toes and cuboid.

*Photographs courtesy Paul Brand, Seattle, USA

cool area and of the hot spot. The difference between the two (we call it the Delta Temperature) indicates the level of inflammation at the hot spot, and thus the danger of breakdown. If a succession of such evening measurements shows a daily increase of the Delta temp., this means that the hot spot will ulcerate if the amount of walking is not reduced until the Delta temperature becomes steady, day after day.

Note that during miles of running, the sensation of pain from commencing traumatic inflammation has made this man change his gait to spare the medial side and shift to the lateral side of his foot. We checked his foot the next day and found that there was tenderness only in the second toe and under the cuboid at the lateral edge of the foot.

If the same run had been with insensitive feet, there would have been no shift of high temperature to the lateral side, and the medial side and great toe would have become intensely hot and might have started to blister.

CLINICAL IMPLICATIONS of Biomechanics

Every attempt should be made to reduce the plantar pressure so as to prevent foot ulceration. In-shoe measurement of plantar pressure has revealed that it can be reduced by more than 50% by extra depth and cushioning of the footwear. Plantar pressure analysis can help refine the assessment of patient risk and give important information for footwear prescription. Accomodation of foot deformities in extra depth shoes with high toe box, cushioned or molded insoles, to redistribute plantar pressure, will help in reducing the risk of plantar ulceration. Patients with high plantar pressures should reduce their activity level, walk slowly with short steps and take adequate care of feet. The footcare team should analyse and closely monitor areas of high plantar pressure. In addition there should be regular removal of the callus and bulk of the thickened nails. The goals of treatment should be to reduce the risk of primary foot ulceration and recurrence in those with previous ulceration.

Following references have been referred for technical information in this chapter.
- Peter R. Cavanagh, Jan S. Ulbrecht and Gregory M. Caputo. The Biomechanics of the Foot in Diabetes Mellitus. In Levin and O'Neal's. The Diabetic foot. John H. Bowker, Michael A Pfeifer eds. Mosby Year Book Inc.; 2001, 125-196.
- Paul Brand. Insensitive Feet. A practical handbook on foot problems in leprosy. The Leprosy Mission, London : 1981.

4 Great Toe

It is apt to call it "Great toe"
rather than calling it "Big toe"

The great toe is the widest and longest of all the toes with the second toe having equal length in many individuals. It has two phalanges unlike other toes which have three. Two sesamoid bones are always present in the tendons of flexor hallucis brevis, on the plantar aspect of the metatarsophalangeal joint of the hallux and are firmly tied in the medial part of the plantar aponeurosis (Fig. 4.1). Although their precise functions are not known, these help to modify plantar pressure, diminish friction, and alter the direction of pull of a muscle.

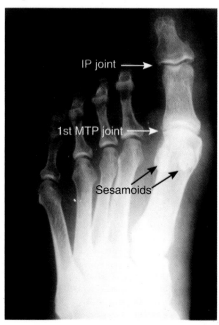

Fig. 4.1: Radiograph of the foot, note a strong 1st ray with its metatarsal, two phalanges and two sesamoids

In midstance, the great toe along with its metatarsal (first ray) bears about a third of body weight and during the toe-off phase, the head of the first metatarsal endures maximum body weight. The first metatarsal along with two lateral metatarsals form the anterior part of the medial arch. We all know from our anatomy days that the thumb is the most important among all the fingers of the hand and it is said that if the thumb is lost, fifty percent of hand function is lost. The thumb has several movements, flexion, extension, adduction, abduction, and opposition. It carries out skilled movements alongwith other fingers. This dexterity of the hand distinguishes us from the rest of the animal kingdom. On the other hand, the great toe has known only two movements, flexion and extension. However, with its metatarsal, it contributes tremendously in weight bearing, propulsion, stability of the foot, and maintaining the medial arch of the foot. Rightly so, this significance has not escaped the surgeons, who would much rather preserve the first ray, even in the face of sacrificing the four lateral rays. If the great toe is infected, the surgeon will try to preserve the proximal portion by carrying out amputation at the interphalangeal joint (IP) and as a last resort would go for metatarsophalangeal (MTP) disarticulation. Even if the first metatarsal is involved, the surgeon would endeavour to preserve atleast a part of it, for sake of foot stability. Despite its enormous contribution, the heroic acts of the great toe go unsung.

In neuropathic foot lesions however, the great toe is frequently involved in the disease process. The majority of advanced neuropathic foot lesions originate from the great toe with more than forty percent of plantar ulcers being situated either on the ball of the great toe or head of the first metatarsal (Fig. 4.2, 4.3).

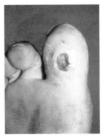

Fig. 4.2:   Ulcer on the ball of the great toe

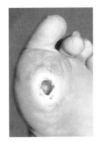

Fig. 4.3:   Ulcer on 1st MT head.

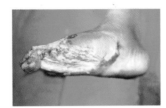

Fig. 4.4: Great toe infection spreading along the tendon sheaths

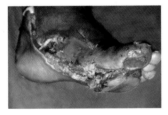

Fig. 4.5: Great toe infection spreading proximally into the leg

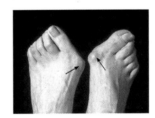

Fig. 4.6: Hallux valgus, note risk areas on prominent MT heads

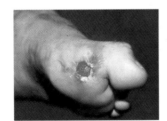

Fig. 4.7:   Cock-up deformity with plantar ulceration

Infection in the great toe can rapidly spread along the tendon sheaths of its two long muscles, the extensor hallucis longus and the flexor hallucis longus (Fig.4.4, 4.5). The great toe is vulnerable to trauma and a majority of nail lesions (paronychia, nail dystrophies) find house in it. Limited joint mobility afflicts the great toe significantly (hallux rigidus) as do deformities such as cocked-up toe and hallux valgus (Fig. 4.6, 4.7).

Diabetic neuropathy probably originates and is at its worst in the great toe. It is probably a length related neuropathy; the great toe being farthest structure in the human body requires the longest nerves. This could be one of the reasons why foot lesions commonly occur in the great toe.

No wonder that in prevention of diabetic foot, and particularly the neuropathic one, the great toe fetches a meticulous and that much closer look. So, as it would seem, it is much more than just being a case of 'size matters'.

Case study (4.A)

This 55 year old male with type 2 DM, of only 3 months duration, presented with non healing wound of the right great toe. He had sustained thermal injury (silencer burn) three months ago following which he developed discoloration of the great toe. He was being treated elsewhere with insulin, antibiotics and dressings for the wound. On examination, he had neuropathy, normal ABI and gangrenous changes with destruction of the great toe (Fig. 4.8 A). He was hospitalized, switched on to intravenous antibiotics, intensified insulin therapy and was subjected to **disarticulation at the 1st MTP joint** and the wound was closed primarily. The wound healed completely in four weeks (Fig. 4.8 B). He was advised about footcare and preventive footwear.

Prolonged contact with hot surface can lead to deep burns, if the wound is not debrided in time, it gets secondarily infected leading to destruction of the soft tissues and deeper structures as happened in this case.

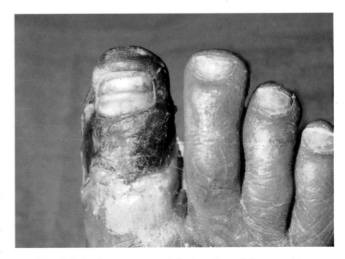

Fig. 4.8 A: Gangrene and destruction of the great toe

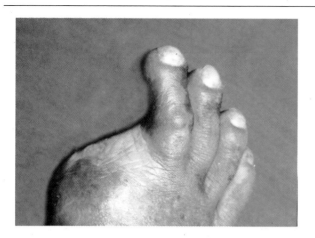

Fig. 4.8 B: Disarticulation at 1st MTP joint

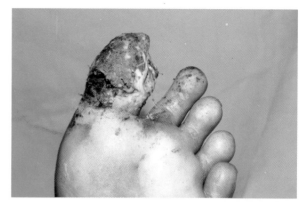

Fig. 4.9A: Herbs packed in the wound

Case study (4.B)

This 64 year old male with type 2 DM of 16 years duration, presented with nonhealing wound of left great toe for six weeks. His general and systemic examinations were normal. He had neuropathic feet with normal ABI. There was swelling over the dorsum and the great toe was found to be completely packed with paste of herbs (Fig. 4.9 A) which had to be removed with great efforts. The great toe was totally destroyed (Fig.4.9 B), however the plantar aspect of the foot was apparently normal. X-ray of the foot revealed osteomyelitis of the phalanges of the great toe.

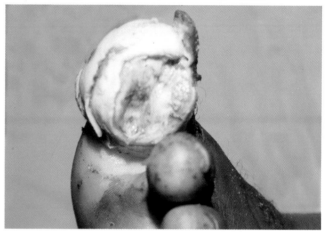

Fig. 4.9B: Destroyed great toe

He was hospitalized and switched on to intravenous antibiotics, intensified insulin therapy and was posted for disarticulation of the great toe. However, during surgery, it was seen that there was gross necrosis of the deeper tissues of the foot including muscles and tendons; (Fig.4.9 C) the surgeon realized that disarticulating the great toe alone was not the solution and after obtaining a fresh consent, a **below knee amputation** was carried out. The bacterial swab taken during surgery later on revealed growth of *Pseudomonas aeruginosa*.

Infected diabetic foot is a tricky situation and it is often difficult to assess clinically the anatomical extent of the infective process. Clinically it had not appeared that this patient would require such a radical ampu-

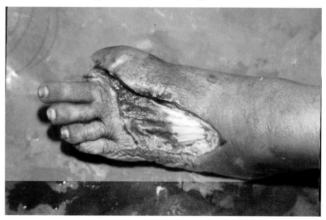

Fig. 4.9C: On debridement, necrosis of deep tissues noted in the foot.

tation. Packing the wound with herbs might have further worsened the wound.

5   Heel

Heel ulcers do not heal easily!

Heel is the toughest part of the foot. 'Heel strike', when the foot first touches the ground, is the very first thing during the gait cycle and here most of the body weight is borne by the heel bone (calcaneus). However, at that stage the other foot is still sharing some of the weight of the body. As soon as the heel is firmly on the ground the other foot leaves the ground and then for a moment the calcaneus may carry the whole body weight. The skin of the heel is tightly bound by numerous vertical septa extending through the subcutaneous tissue to the surface of the calcaneus. These septa result in formation of small cylinders which are packed with fat globules. During weight bearing, each fat globule changes its shape and spreads the thrust to the globules on either side as well as to those immediately below it. Thus by the time that thrust gets down to the skin it is not a small area but rather a large area that is carrying weight (Fig. 5.1). These peculiar fatty cylinders act like shock absorbers which is why, in Syme's amputation, the heel flap is preserved for weight bearing even though the calcaneus is removed.

Despite increased plantar pressure on the heel during walking, neuropathic plantar ulcers are less common on the heel as compared to the forefoot. The possible explanations are that the bony prominences of the forefoot are not covered by subcutaneous tissue as thick as the heel and secondly loss of protective

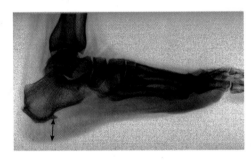

Fig. 5.1: Radiograph showing strong calcaneus with its thick heel pad (soft tissue shadow)

sensibility is greater in the forefoot with the longest nerve fibers preferentially affected.

HEEL LESIONS

Fissures, Infections, Friction Injuries

Fissures are a common feature on the borders of the heel and are deep and wide (Fig. 5.2). These result from dry skin, a consequence of autonomic neuropathy, can be very deep and can get secondarily infected. The heel is particularly vulnerable to trauma. Associated neuropathy leads to callus building as the heel is exposed to a great deal of pressure. Regular removal of such callus is essential (Fig. 5.3, 5.4). Lesions of the posterior portion of the heel usually indicate excessive walking with tight footwear on the insensate foot (Fig. 5.5). When the site of deep ulceration and

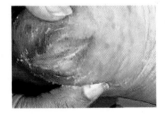

Fig. 5.2: Fissure on the heel border

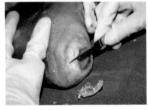

Fig. 5.3: Heel ulcer, callus being removed

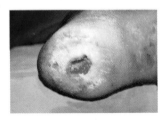

Fig. 5.4: After callus removal, note healing ulcer

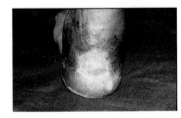

Fig. 5.5: Heel ulcer over posterior portion (friction injury)

gangrene happens to be heel (Fig. 5.6), the foot is seldom salvageable because debridement and amputations in this area often preclude functional weight bearing. The heel may also get secondarily involved with infection spread from the forefoot or mid foot in the deep plantar layer (Fig. 5.7). Heel involvement and osteomyelitis of the calcaneus (Fig. 5.8) are often intractable surgical problems. Lower limb amputation is often necessary.

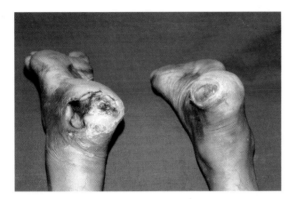
Fig. 5.6: Gangrene of the heel right, ulcer on left

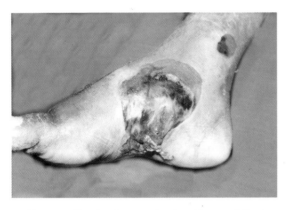
Fig. 5.7: Proximal spread to heel from midfoot

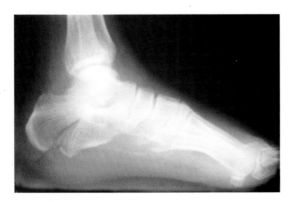
Fig. 5.8: Osteomyelitis of the calcaneus

Ischemic Ulcer

The heel is supplied by the posterior tibial artery and this is often occluded in diabetics. In any heel ulcer which is not healing (Fig. 5.9), disease of the posterior tibial artery must be looked for. Such a vulnerable foot may be salvaged if vascular reconstruction is offered in time.

Decubitus Ulcer

When a patient requires prolonged bed rest, particular attention must be paid to the heels. Because of loss of sensibility the patient tends to keep the heels in the same position, which results in pressure necrosis (Fig. 5.10). The skin breaks down and infection and gangrene can develop (Fig. 5.11). The simple weight

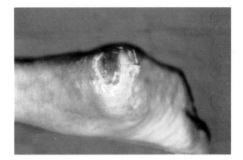
Fig. 5.9: Ischemic ulcer on the heel

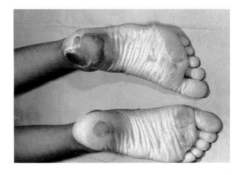
Fig. 5.10: Decubitus ulcers

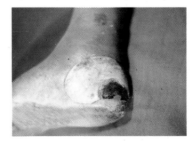
Fig. 5.11: Decubitus ulcer with gangrene

of the immobile foot on the mattress obliterates blood perfusion in skin on the posterolateral side of the heel. The degree of vulnerability of the debilitated foot is often not appreciated by the patient and even the physician, who may have difficulty in understanding why "such a little thing" can result in tissue loss with consequences as grave as leg amputation. Prevention is thus the heart of the matter. All this makes for three simple take home messages. Daily inspection of heels in bedridden patients, frequently turning the patient, and the mandatory use of heel protectors (Fig. 5.12). Sadly, it is the simple that is often ignored.

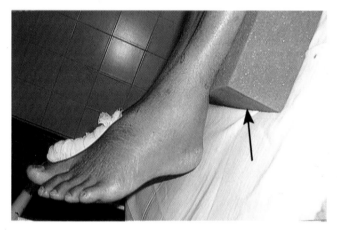

Fig. 5.12: Heel protector

Case Study (5.A)

This 56 year male with type 2 DM of 11 years, presented with non healing wounds over both heels since 8 weeks. History revealed that he had dryness of plantar skin and deep fissures over both heels. Intense itching compelled him to peel off the everted skin over the fissures which bled. The patient noticed swelling over both heels after 2 days. He received antibiotics and dressings were carried out, but the ulcers continued to discharge purulent material. His general physical and systemic examinations were normal. He had neuropathic feet with normal ABI. The wounds were not deep and the X-ray of both feet did not reveal evidence of osteomyelitis. He was subjected to surgical debridement. After removal of the necrotic tissue, the edges of the right foot wound were approximated and primary suturing carried out. The left foot wound was cleaned and split skin grafting

carried out 1 week after the appearance of red granulation tissue (Fig. 5.13).

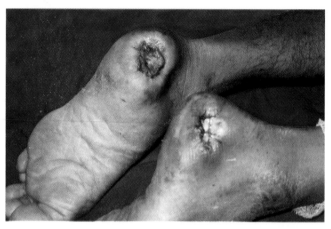

Fig. 5.13: Bilateral heel ulcers healed, right, after suturing and left with a skin graft

The patient was advised to wear protective footwear and apply emollients to prevent dryness. The fissures are wide and deep in neuropathic feet and can easily ulcerate and pave way for microorganisms, leading to a limb threatening situation.

Case Study (5.B)

This 57 year old male with type 2 DM of 15 years, presented with nonhealing wound left foot since two months. History revealed that he had deep fissures over the heel which were infected secondarily. He was treated elsewhere with antibiotics and insulin and the surgical debridement was carried out. Despite surgery the wound did not heal and the patient continued to get fever and discharge from wound. His general and systemic examinations were normal except for hypertension. Local examination revealed that he had neuropathic feet with normal ABI. He had deep heel pad infection with areas of necrosis and slough (Fig. 5.14 A).

He was hospitalized and switched on to intensified insulin therapy, intravenous antibiotics. His investigations revealed Hb 8 gms%, TLC 10,500/cu.mm, ESR 141/1st hr, S. Creatinine 1.2 mg%, plasma glucose of 283 mg% and HbA$_1$c 9.2%. X-ray of the foot did not reveal any evidence of osteomyelitis. His resting ECG showed old anteroseptal myocardial infarction, 2D echocardiograph showed an ejection

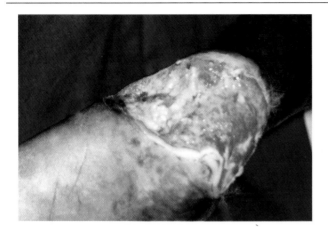

Fig. 5.14A: Infected heel pad

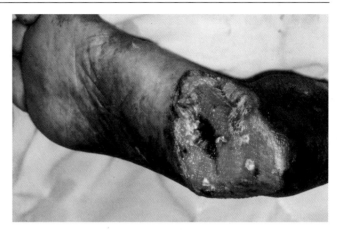

Fig. 5.14B: After debridement

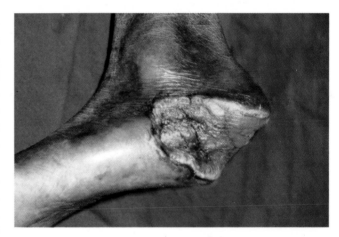

Fig. 5.14C: After a skin graft

fraction of 45% and diastolic dysfunction. A cardiologist was consulted who initiated the appropriate treatment. In view of non healing heel pad infection, old myocardial infarction, a duplex Doppler of the left leg arterial system was carried out especially, to find out the status of the posterior tibial artery which is the dominant artery for blood supply to heel pad. It revealed triphasic wave form, patent posterior tibial, and other infrapopliteal vessels.

He was subjected to surgical debridement and necrotic tissue and slough were removed. A bacterial swab was sent for culture and sensitivity, which revealed a scanty growth of *Streptococcus pyogens*. The wound was regularly dressed with complete immobilization of the left lower limb. Three weeks later, after appearance of healthy granulation tissue, the wound was closed with a split skin graft (Fig. 5.14B, 5.14C). The deep heel pad infection had left a significant defect in the heel. The patient was gradually mobilised and given heel relief shoes with weight bearing mainly on forefoot and midfoot. He was advised to use the feet sparingly (Fig.5.14D).

Heel pad infection is a difficult surgical problem and being abundant in fatty tissue, infection can lead to fat necrosis as there is no intervening red muscle mass, and can easily spread into the calcaneus. In this case fortunately, there was no osteomyelitis of the calcaneus, and the posterior tibial artery was not diseased. Hence the limb salvage was possible.

Case Study (5.C)

This 44 year old male with type 2 DM since 14 years, mentally subnormal since childhood, presented with

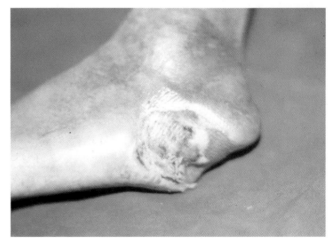

Fig. 5.14D: Six months later

nonhealing ulcer over right heel since six months. His general and systemic examinations were normal and he had neuropathic feet with normal ABI. He had a deep burrowing ulcer over right heel with purulent

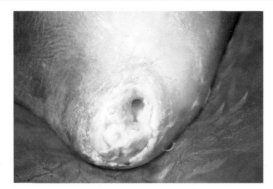

Fig. 5.15A: Deep burrowing heel ulcer

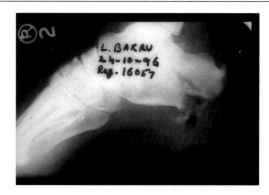

Fig. 5.15B: Osteomyelitis of the calcaneus

discharge (Fig.5.15 A). The ulcer was 2 inch (5 cm) deep and the bone could be probed through the ulcer. His investigations revealed Hb of 10gm%, TLC 12000/cu.mm., ESR 124 mm/1st hr. X-ray of the foot revealed osteomyelitis of the calcaneus (Fig. 5.15 B). Despite higher intravenous antibiotics and improved glycemic control, the wound continued to show signs of deterioration. The patient eventually required **below knee amputation.**

Heel pad infection with osteomyelitis of calcaneus are often intractable surgical problems. A leg amputation is often necessary. This patient's mental subnormality aggravated the problem further because of non compliance.

6 Examination of Feet

All that you need is a pair of sensible hands and eyes

Examination of feet is an integral part of physical examination of every patient, more so a diabetic patient. The goal should be to identify :
- Normal feet
- Feet at risk
- Presence of significant neuropathy
- Presence of significant ischemia
- Presence of foot lesions

Screening procedure should be quantifiable, reproducible, predictive and inexpensive.

Inspection

The examiner should insist on removal of the shoes and socks or stockings even if the patient is reluctant, as it is not uncommon to see an active ulcer or even gangrenous changes, of which the patient is totally ignorant. One should look for neuropathic changes (Fig. 6.1) like dry skin, fissures, deformities, callus, abnormal shape of foot, ulceration, prominent veins, and nail lesions. A careful attention should be given to the interdigital spaces (Fig. 6.2). A significant ischemia is characterized by loss of hair on the dorsum

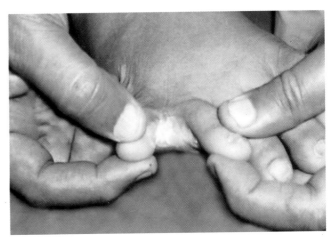

Fig. 6.2: Maceration in the interdigital space

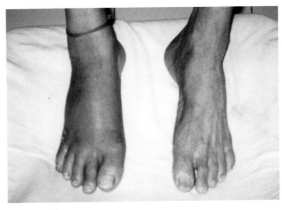

Fig. 6.3: Dependent rubor, right foot

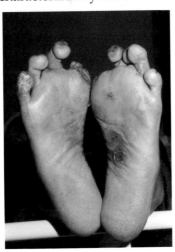

Fig. 6.1: Feet showing neuropathic changes

of foot and a dependent rubor (Fig. 6.3). I always use a mirror to show the patient his/her plantar surface as most of them have not seen it for ages. The inspection of feet should be done at every clinic visit.

Palpation

Touching someone's feet is a sign of highest respect in an Indian culture. The patient realizes the importance of his feet when the doctor touches them.

One should feel whether the foot is warm or cold, examine the peripheral pulsations like dorsalis pedis, which can be felt lateral to the extensor hallucis longus tendon, and the posterior tibial, which is above and behind the medial malleolus. The femoral artery should also be palpated and auscultated for the presence of bruit. The plantar aspects of the feet should be felt for presence of any bony prominences.

Examination of Footwear

The majority of diabetics do not need special footwear, at the same time it should not be ill fitting or tight. It should have a broad toe box, a heel height of 5 cm or less and the heel counter should be stiff enough to prevent excessive movement of the foot within the shoe. Those patients who do not like to wear shoes should be advised to wear sandals with velcro and a heel counter. Chappals and "Hawaii" slippers with a grip between the great toe and the second toe should be discouraged. One should also inspect the footwear for signs of wear especially on the outsole (Fig. 6.4). The footwear should not have any protruding objects inside, the uppers should have a soft lining and the insole should be soft. Further details are given in the separate chapter on footwear (see chapter 42).

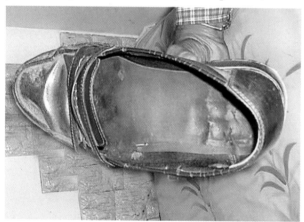

Fig. 6.4: Wornout shoe

Assessment of Significant Neuropathy

Distal symmetric polyneuropathy involves both small and large nerve fibers. Rarely a selective involvement of the small nerve fibers is seen in diabetics such as in painful neuropathy, where selectively the thermal sensation (small nerve fibers) is lost with preservation of touch and vibration (large nerve fibers).

Table 6.1: Nerve fiber functions	
Small nerve fiber	*Large nerve fiber*
Thermal sensation (heat and cold perception) Pain sensation Sweating (sympathetic)	Vibration perception Touch sensation Position sense Deep tendon reflexes Motor nerves.

The sensory neuropathy can be tested by using monofilaments and biothesiometry. If these are not available, the detection of light touch by cotton wool, pinprick and vibration sense using a 128 Hz tuning fork will suffice. The goal is to detect whether the patient has lost protective sensations (LOPS), rendering him susceptible to foot ulceration.

Testing with Monofilament

Nylon monofilament of 5.07 size (thickness), equivalent of 10 gm of linear force should be used. It tests sense of touch (large nerve fiber function). When applied perpendicular to the foot, it buckles at a given force of 10 g (Fig. 6.5, 6.6). The patient should be able to sense the monofilament by the time it buckles. The filament should be pressed at several sites e.g. plantar aspects of the first toe, the first, third, and fifth metatarsal heads, the heel, and dorsum of the foot. The patient's inability to feel the filament indicates a loss of protective sensation (a high-risk foot).

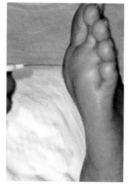

Fig. 6.5: Touching with the monofilament

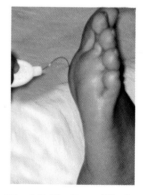

Fig. 6.6: Testing while the monofilament buckles

Biothesiometry

The degree of neuropathy can be further quantified by the use of the biothesiometer (Fig. 6.7). When applied to the foot, it delivers a vibratory stimulus, which increases as the voltage is raised. The biothesio-

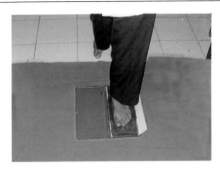

Fig. 6.9: Footprint being taken
on an ink mat

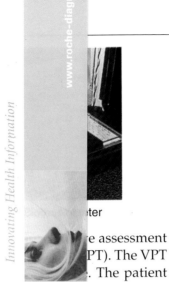

...ter

...e assessment
...PT). The VPT
... The patient
can be classified as a low-risk with VPT<15V, an
intermediate risk with VPT between 16 to 24 V, and a
high-risk with VPT> 25V.

Testing for Ischemia in Foot:
Ankle/Brachial Pressure Index (ABI)

A hand-held Doppler can be used to confirm the
presence of pulses and to quantify the vascular supply
(Fig. 6.8). When used together with a sphygmomanometer, the ankle and brachial systolic pressures can
be measured and the ratio then calculated. In normal
subjects, the ankle systolic pressure is higher than
brachial systolic pressure. The normal ABI is > 1, in
the presence of ischemia it is < 0.9. Absent or feeble
pulses with ABI < 0.9 confirms ischemia. Conversely,
the presence of pulses and ABI > 1 rules out significant
ischemia.

Ink is applied on the other side of the mat, with the
roller. While interpreting the footprint, darker area
indicates a high pressure point (Fig.6.10). This test is
however not quantitative and has its limitations. A
quantitative measurement of plantar pressure is now
available for a barefoot, as well as in-shoe, using a
computer and special software (Fig. 6.11). However
being expensive, it cannot be made available at every
centre.

Once the patient has been classified into either non
risk or high risk category, a further evaluation
depending upon the risk category can be carried out.

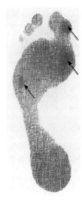

Fig. 6.10: Footprint, darker areas
indicate high pressure points

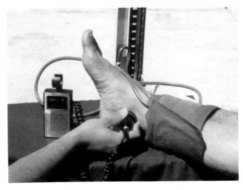

Fig. 6.8: Measuring ankle systolic pressure
with hand-held Doppler

Testing for High Pressure Points

The feet can be evaluated for high pressure points by
a simple inexpensive technique using an ink mat. The
patient is asked to stand or walk on the mat (Fig. 6.9).

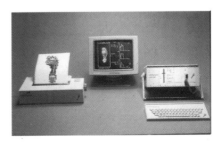

Fig. 6.11: Quantitative measure-ment of
plantar pressure using a computer and
special software

7 Classification and Staging

Some day yet, the ideal classification should ring the bell

A standard classification of the diabetic foot is useful to assess the etiology and prognosis, to facilitate an appropriate treatment, to help monitor the progress, and to serve as a means of communication in a uniform terminology. Although various classifications have been suggested, there is, as yet, no universally acceptable classification. The diabetic foot is classified, as per the underlying etiology, into

- **Neuropathic foot** (Neuropathy is dominant)
- **Neuroischemic foot** (Occlusive vascular disease is dominant)

The presence of infection is of paramount importance as it alters the prognosis adversely and hastens the progress towards a limb amputation. It is therefore extremely important to include its presence or absence in any classification of the diabetic foot.

Suggested Classification

- **Neuropathic foot**
  - a. with infection
  - b. without infection
- **Neuroischemic foot**
  - a. with infection
  - b. without infection

A neuropathic foot can lead to fissures, bullae, callus, edema, digital necrosis, Charcot foot, and plantar ulcers. A neuroischemic foot can lead to pain at rest, ulcerations on the foot margins, digital necrosis, and eventually extensive gangrene. Differentiating between these two entities is essential because their complications are different and they require different therapeutic strategies. For example, digital necrosis in a neuropathic foot often requires just a toe disarticulation and debridement, while a digital necrosis in neuroischemic foot may require a vascular reconstruction and partial amputation, or even a leg amputation, if vascular reconstruction is not feasible.

A purely ischemic foot, with no concomittant neuropathy is rarely seen in diabetic patients and its management remains the same as a neuroischemic foot. The foot lesions can also occur in diabetics without neuropathy or ischemia (non neuroischemic foot). Such foot lesions are secondary to trauma and are invariably infected because of underlying, uncontrolled and often undetected diabetes.

Wagner Classification

It is the most widely quoted classification of diabetic foot (Wagner and Meggitt 1970). It grades the foot into

Table 7.1: Differentiating features between neuropathic and neuroischemic foot (Fig. 7.1, 7.2)		
Characteristics	*Neuropathic Foot*	*Neuroischemic Foot*
Skin temperature	Warm	Cold
Pain	Painless	Painful
Skin colour	Not altered	Dependent rubor
Callus	Thick at pressure points	May or may not be present
Ulcer	Plantar at pressure points Dorsal at areas of stress	Margins of toe
Peripheral pulses	Bounding	Feeble or not palpable
ABI	> 0.9	< 0.9

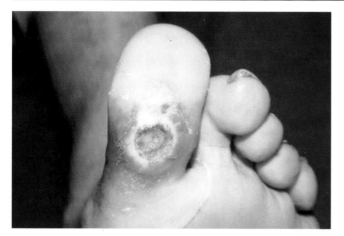

Fig. 7.1: Neuropathic ulcer

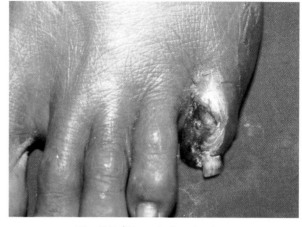

Fig. 7.2: Neuroischemic ulcer

six grades depending upon the severity of lesion. However, the perfusion of foot and neuroarthropathy (Charcot foot) are not duely considered in this classification.

Every diabetic foot lesion does not have to necessarily go through all these stages. For example in a neuroischemic foot, the presenting lesion could skip from a grade 1 to grade 4 without passing through the intermediate grades. The goal of management should be to reverse the grade although this is seldom possible except for grade 1 to 3.

Wagner Classification

Grade 0 :

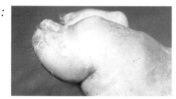

Fig. 7.3: No ulceration in a high-risk foot

Grade 1 :

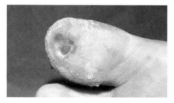

Fig. 7.4: Superficial ulceration

Grade 2 :

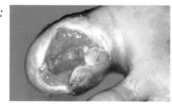

Fig. 7.5: Deep ulceration that penetrates to the tendon, bone or joint

Grade 3 :

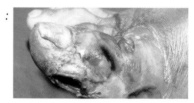

Fig. 7.6: Osteomyelitis or a deep abscess

Grade 4 :

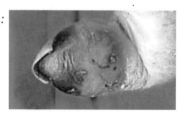

Fig. 7.7: Localized gangrene

Grade 5 :

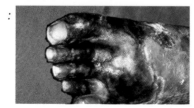

Fig. 7.8: Extensive gangrene requiring a major amputation

Depth-ischemia Classification

It is a modification of the Wagner classification, and is used in the following manner. Each foot is graded with both, a number and a letter. The combination of the two describes the physical extent of the wound (number) and the presence or absence of ischemia (letter).

A. No ischemia

B. Ischemia without gangrene

Grades C and D are almost same as grades 4 and 5 of the Wagner classification. Thus Wagner grades 0, 1, 2 and 3 can be re-classified by the addition of a letter A or B depending upon the presence or absence of ischemia.

Staging a Diabetic Foot

The natural history of diabetic foot can be divided into six stages (ME Edmonds and AVM Foster). Most diabetic foot problems fall under one of the six stages (Fig.7.9 to 7.14). The exceptions being the Charcot foot and pathological fractures.

Stage	Clinical Condition	Stage	Clinical Condition

Stage   **Clinical Condition**

1.

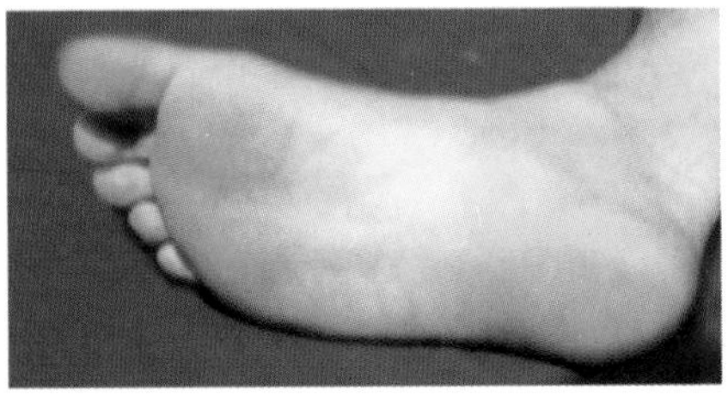

Fig. 7.9: Normal

2.

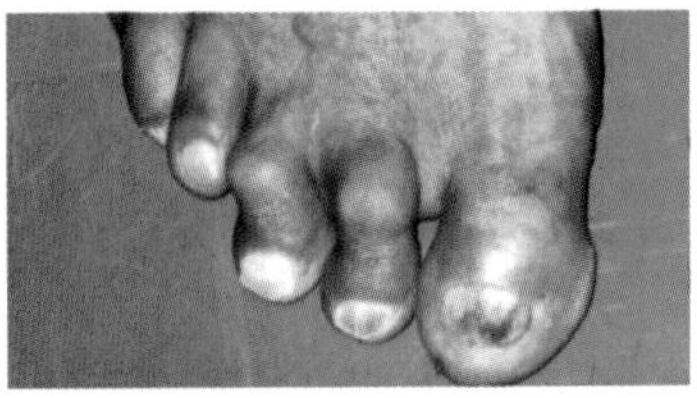

Fig. 7.10: High-risk

3.

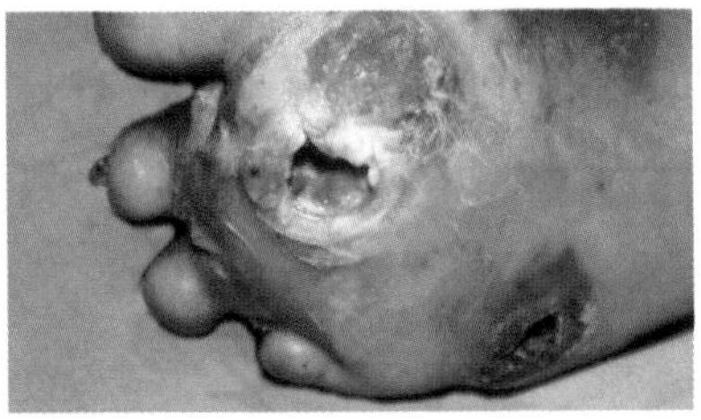

Fig. 7.11: Ulcerated

Stage   **Clinical Condition**

4.

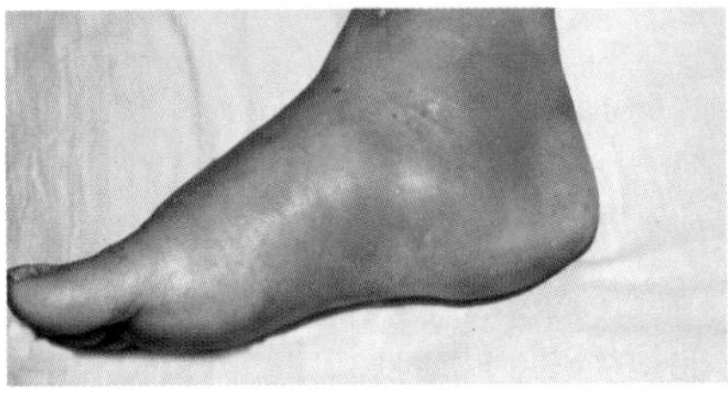

Fig. 7.12: Cellulitic

5.

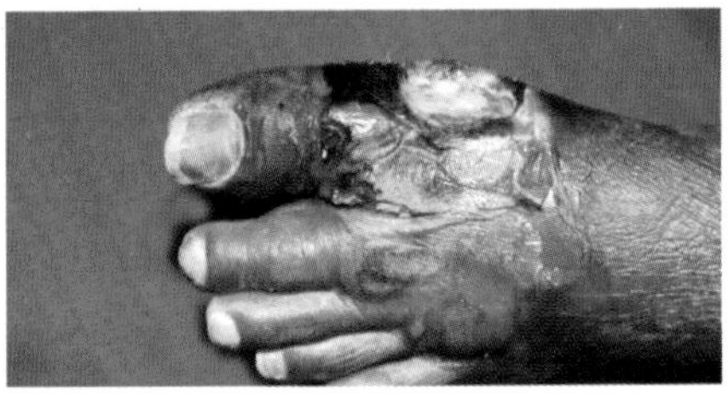

Fig. 7.13: Necrotic

6.

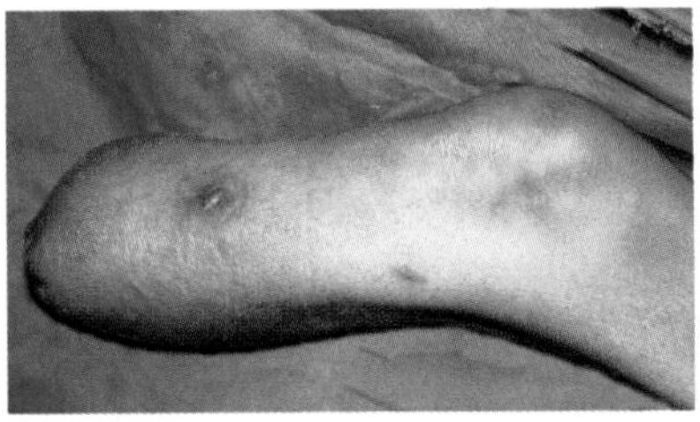

Fig. 7.14: Major amputation

The most important feature, which everyone involved in the care of a diabetic foot needs to know are whether

a. The foot is neuropathic or neuroischemic

b. It is infected or not

The prognosis, evaluation and the management differ significantly upon these factors.

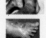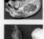

8 Etiopathogenesis of Neuropathic Ulcers

Plantar ulcers do not occur overnight
Damage begins inside the foot and surface afterwards
— Price

Diabetic foot ulcers occur in approximately 4% to 10% of patients. It is important to realize that 85% of all diabetic amputations are preceded by foot ulcers, thus making it extremely important to understand the pathogenesis of foot ulceration and strategies to heal them. Preservation of intact skin is very essential. Following are the various risk factors associated with diabetic foot ulcerations :

Primary Risk Factors

- Significant polyneuropathy with loss of protective sensations
- Evidence of ischemia in foot (ABI < 0.9)

Secondary Risk Factors

- Foot deformities
- Callus
- Previous ulcer
- Previous amputation
- Chronic renal failure
- Inappropriate footwear
- Impaired vision
- Person living alone
- Low educational status
- Non compliant patient.

Table 8.1 : Causative factors for neuropathic ulcers

Extrinsic factors	Intrinsic factors
Ill fitting footwear	Limited joint mobility
Barefoot walking	Bony prominences
Falls/accidents	Foot deformities
Objects inside shoes	Neuro-arthropathy
Thermal trauma	Plantar callus
Injury by sharp objects	Scar tissue
Home surgery	Fissures

Neuropathic foot ulcerations frequently result from two or more risk factors occuring together. In diabetic polyneuropathy all the nerve fibers are affected (sensory, motor and autonomic), which leaves the foot with loss of protective sensations (LOPS). Any damaging stimuli or external trauma are either perceived less or not at all, resulting in an ulcer. **Sensory neuropathy is the most important prerequisite for foot ulcerations.** All the other factors contribute to foot ulceration only in the presence of sensory neuropathy.

Motor neuropathy leads to atrophy and weakness of the intrinsic muscles of the foot (intrinsic minus foot), results in clawed toes and an abnormal walking pattern. The fibrofatty tissues which act like cushions for metatarsal heads (metatarsal cushions), are pushed forward due to deformities, leading to an increased pressure on the metatarsal heads (Fig. 8.1). Autonomic neuropathy results in reduced or absent sweating causing plantar xerosis with cracks and fissures. Limited joint mobility, foot deformities and abnormal gait result in an altered biomechanical loading of the foot with elevated plantar foot pressures and probably

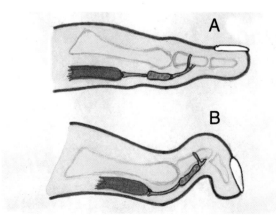

Fig. 8.1A and B: **(A)** Normal position of fibrofatty tissue **(B)** Fibrofatty tissue pushed forward

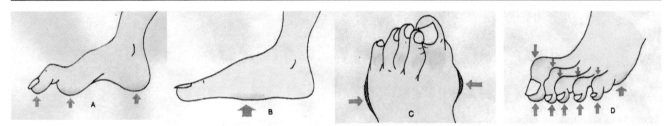

Fig. 8.2A to D: Showing areas of high-risk for foot ulceration
(Reproduced by kind permission by the "International Working Group on the Diabetic Foot")

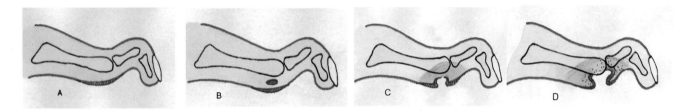

Fig. 8.3: Stages of plantar ulcer A - Callus, B - Soft tissue damage, C - Ulceration, D -Infection.
(Reproduced with kind permission of the "International Working Group on the Diabetic Foot")

increased shear forces (Fig. 8.2). Loss of protective sensations coupled with the repetitive trauma of walking, in presence of raised plantar pressures, results in a plantar callus. Growth of plantar callus further increases the local skin pressure as it works as a foreign body on the skin surface (Fig. 8.3). Neuropathic foot ulceration results from factors extrinsic to insensitive foot such as an external trauma, often together with intrinsic factors such as increased plantar pressure. These intrinsic and extrinsic factors are discussed individually in subsequent chapters.

Plantar ulcers do not occur overnight but are a result of repetitive stress of walking and abnormal weight bearing, resulting in chronic tissue damage.

9

Sharp Injuries

Speaking bluntly, sharps can harm like hell

Painless mechanical trauma can occur from a variety of causes. Barefoot walking with normal sensations rarely results in an injury and that is precisely the reason why normal sensations are called protective sensations. Walking barefoot with loss of protective sensations is however an open invitation for injury. A person with normal sensations will stop as soon as he feels a thorn prick and would not take even one more step until the thorn is removed. If he continues to walk after pulling out the thorn, he will walk unevenly with the painful part of his foot kept off the ground. However, the person with loss of protective sensations, does not even know that he has a thorn prick and goes on walking. The thorn gets driven deeper into his foot carrying infection with it. (Fig. 9.1).

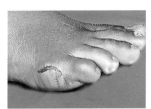 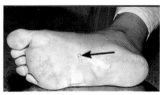

Fig. 9.2: Glass prick injury

Fig. 9.3: Nail prick injury to midfoot, wound discharging pus

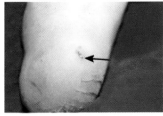 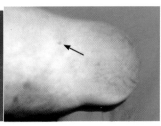

Fig. 9.4: Stone pieces stuck close to left heal

Fig. 9.5: Wooden splinter stuck close to heel (patient was not aware of it)

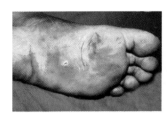 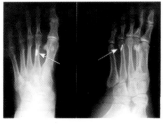

Fig. 9.6: Thorn prick close to heel

Fig. 9.7: Radiograph A P and oblique views showing foreign body probably a nail

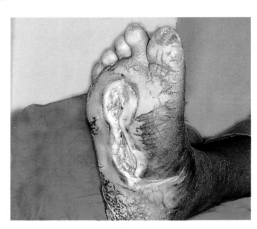

Fig. 9.1: Severely infected foot secondary to sharp injury

SHARP OBJECTS

Stepping unknowingly on sharp objects like a thorn, piece of glass, nail, or a piece of stone can lead to painless puncture wounds in diabetic neuropathic feet (Fig. 9.2 to 9.7). During a clinic visit it is not uncommon to notice a foreign body usually a wood splinter or a thorn, still stuck in the plantar skin, about which the patient is ignorant. Midfoot is conspicuously the common site for such puncture wounds. There are interesting stories about such puncture wounds cited in the literature or heard during lectures, like a carpenter's nail lodged in the foot for over a month without the patient being aware of it. X-ray of the foot revealed it, but the damage had already occurred and the foot needed amputation. A patient trying hard to remove his shoes failed; his watchful daughter noticed a nail, which had pierced the shoe sole and plantar sole as well. The nail had to be removed first before the shoe.

Home Surgery

Patients are tempted to carry out home surgeries because of absent sensations. The commonly used objects are unsterile shaving blades, razors, needles and pins. Home surgery is another common cause of foot injury. Patients frequently cut their calluses too deep and nails too short resulting in ulcerations. Corn caps and application of salicylic acid can lead to chemical trauma (Fig. 9.8, 9.9).

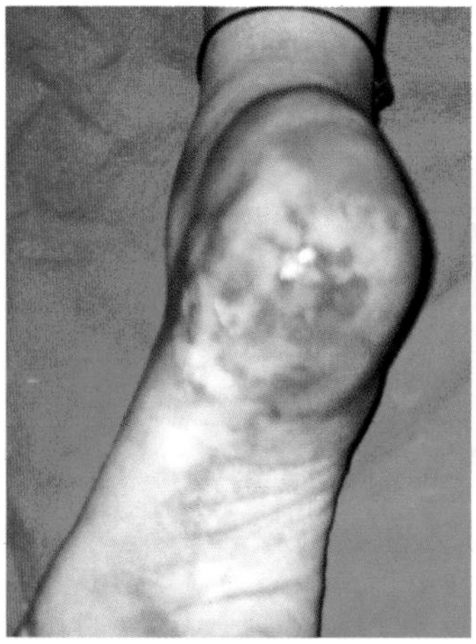

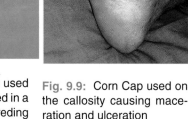

Fig. 9.8: Sewing needle used for home surgery, resulted in a serious heel infection spreding proximally

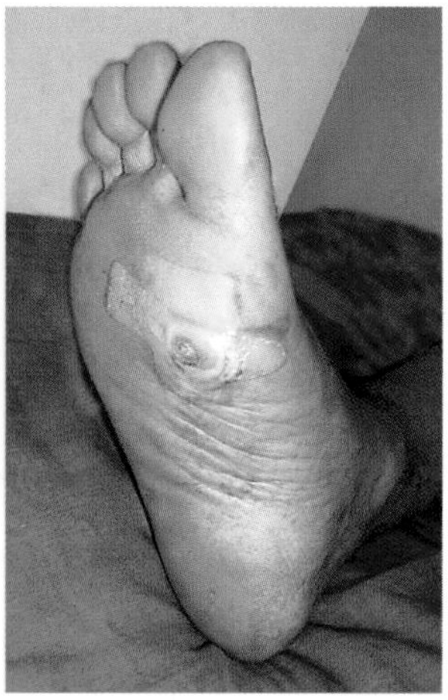

Fig. 9.9: Corn Cap used on the callosity causing maceration and ulceration

Toe Ring Injury

Indian women wear metal toe rings in one or more toes, but commonly in the second toes of both feet (Fig. 9.10). In neuropathic feet with deformities of toes, these toe rings can be a source of injury and can also cause strangulation, if the toe is infected and swollen (Fig. 9.11 to 9.13).

Sharp injuries are often responsible for deadly deep plantar compartment infections, as evident from following cases and cases cited elsewhere in the atlas (Case studies 29.D, 33.B, 39.C, 31.E, 31.F). Repeated instructions, proper education about foot care, and

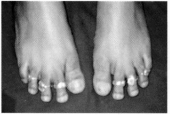 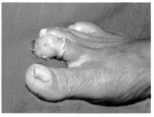

Fig. 9.10: Multiple toe rings in both feet

Fig. 9.11: 2nd toe abscess due to toe ring

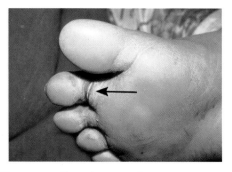

Fig. 9.12: Toe ring causing cut wound on plantar aspect 2nd toe

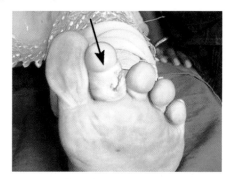

Fig. 9.13: Toe ring causing strangulation of the 2nd toe with ulceration

avoiding barefoot walking can prevent atleast some if not all of these injuries.

Case Study (9.A)

A 55 year old female with type 2 DM of five years had a fall when the toe ring of her right foot got caught in a stone. Next day, she noticed swelling of the foot. Her treating doctor removed the toe ring the next day and punctured a blister. Two days later she had high grade fever with chills and she noticed discoloration of her three toes. She was treated with oral antidiabetics, oral antibiotics, and dressings of the wound done by her family physician. She came to us two weeks later because of increasing swelling and blackening of the toes. Examination of the foot revealed swelling on the dorsum of the right forefoot, necrosis of the 2nd, 3rd and 4th toes with gangrenous changes of the toes and dorsal skin (Fig. 9.14 A, 9.14 B). The plantar aspect revealed swelling and erythema on the middle of the forefoot.

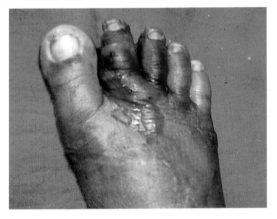

Fig. 9.14A: Swelling of the right foot, gangrene of 2nd to 4th toes with strangulation of 2nd toe

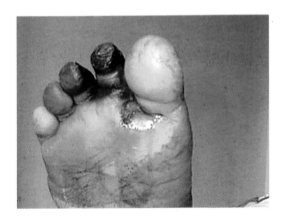

Fig. 9.14B: Showing erythema, swelling on plantar aspect of the foot with gangrene of 2nd to 4th toes

She had evidence of loss of protective sensations in her feet with ABI of >1. Duplex Doppler of the right leg arterial system showed a normal triphasic pattern in all the leg vessels with a suspicion of thrombosis of the plantar arch. She was switched on to intravenous antibiotics, multiple injections of insulin, and was posted for surgery with a tentative diagnosis of plantar abscess over the plantar arch causing the digital necrosis. Under regional anesthesia, the gangrenous toes and the isolated 5th toe alongwith the metatarsal heads were excised. The necrotic material was removed and the gangrenous dorsal skin was excised. Three weeks later, the dorsal skin defect was closed

by a split skin graft and plantar skin was mobilized to cover the cut edges of the metatarsal shafts (Fig. 9.14 C, 9.14 D).

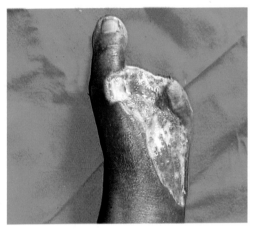

Fig. 9.14C: After radical debridement and amputations of 2nd to 5th toes with MT heads. Great toe being retained

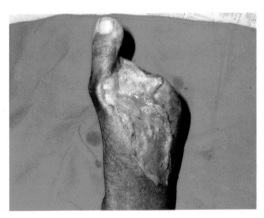

Fig. 9.14D: The wound closed by skin grafting

The great toe was retained to preserve the medial plantar arch and stability of the foot, while the apparently healthy 5th toe was removed as, such an isolated little toe would have lost the support of other toes and would have suffered recurrent trauma.

Case Study (9.B)

This 65 year old male with recent onset type 2 DM, had a nail prick injury in the 2nd webspace of right foot, which was followed by swelling on the dorsum of the foot, associated with dull pain and fever with chills. His treating doctor rightly ordered for plasma glucose estimation which turned out to be 423 mg% and that is how he got referred to our centre. In the meantime, the patient had also consulted a faith healer who tied a holy thread around his ankle assuring him that the infection would not spread beyond the level of the tied thread. On examination he had gross cellulitis on the dorsum with exudative wound in the 2nd web space. He did not have evidence of neuropathy or ischemia (non neuroischemic foot). He underwent surgical debridement with a long incision beginning in the 2nd web space and extending right upto the ankle. The necrotic tissue was debrided and the patient was discharged from the hospital after five days of intravenous antibiotics. He was managed ambulatory on oral antibiotics, dressings and multiple insulin injections. The wound healed in two months though with scarring (Fig. 9.15 A to 9.15 E).

He is one of those few cases where foot lesions have occured secondary to an injury because of underlying, uncontrolled, and undetected DM without neuropathy or ischemia.

Case Study (9.C)

This 56 year old male with type 2 DM of 5 years, presented with fever and swelling of left foot. Fifteen days ago he had sustained sharp injury to the plantar aspect following which, he noticed a gradually increasing swelling and redness. On examination he had neuropathic feet with a normal ABI. He had swelling over left midfoot plantar aspect with yellowish discoloration of the skin surrounded by erythema. He was hospitalized, switched on to intravenous antibiotics, and intensified insulin therapy. X-ray of the foot did not reveal osteomyelitis, gas, or a foreign body. He was subjected to radical wound debridement and **a foreign body (wood splinter)** was removed. The purulent material and necrotic tissue were debrided. Removal of the necrotic plantar skin left a considerable defect, which was later closed by a split skin graft (Fig. 9.16 A, 9.16 B). The patient was advised not to walk barefoot and also to wear appropriate protective footwear.

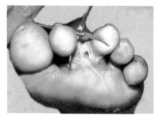 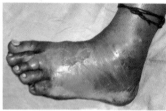

Fig. 9.15A: Sharp injury leading to 2nd web space infection

Fig. 9.15B: Webspace infection with extention into dorsum of the foot

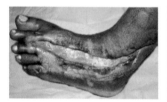 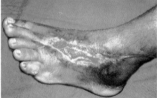

Fig. 9.15C: After debridement

Fig. 9.15D: Healthy granulation tissue

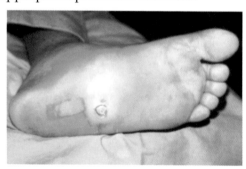

Fig. 9.16A: Midfoot abscess of the left foot, wooden splinter was found inside the wound

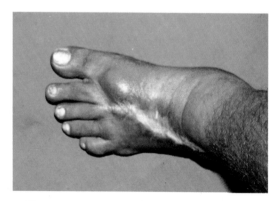

Fig. 9.15E: The wound healed with scarring

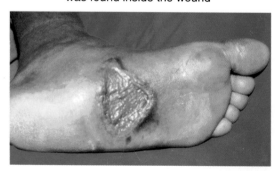

Fig. 9.16B: The wound closed by skin grafting after removal of wooden splinter and thorough debridement

10 Shoe Bite

Of course, protect shoes do, but not infrequently shoes do hurt too

Our feet were originally designed for barefoot walking, but with civilization and modernization, footwear became a necessity. Eversince footwear have come in vogue, majority of the foot problems in normal population have their origin in fancy looking but often faulty footwear. For example, foot deformities (hallux valgus), metatarsalgia, bunious, etc. In persons with diabetes especially with insensate feet, ill-fitting footwear can lead to disastrous foot lesions often requiring amputation.

Ill Fitting Shoes

Injuries from ill fitting shoes are extremely common. Patients with neuropathy invariably wear tight shoes as they do not have any discomfort wearing them. Ulcers caused by ill–fitting shoes occur most often on the margin of toes, behind the heel or on the sides of the foot (Fig. 10.1). In India, open type of footwear (chappals) are commonly worn which have a single grip pattern (Fig. 10.2). These often cause injury over dorsum of the great toe, in the 1st web space and dorsum of the foot (Fig. 10.3 to 10.5). The ulceration is due to pressure ischemia. This pressure is the result of tension within the leather that applies the greatest stress in areas of smallest circumference. This breakdown is also related to the length of time a shoe is worn. Damage occurs when unremitting pressure from a tight shoe is maintained for long hours. Persons with diabetes should be taught not to wear new pair of shoes for a longer duration. They should be instructed to buy shoes preferably in the evening. One should remember the dictum, that the footwear in which foot has ulcerated should never be reused.

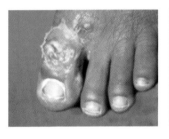

Fig. 10.3: Injury over dorsum of the great toe caused due to footwear such as type A

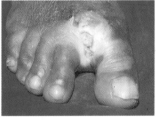

Fig. 10.4: Injury in the 1st web space caused due to footwear such as type B and C

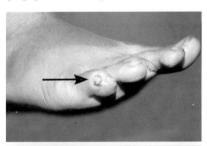

Fig. 10.1: Shoe bite, little toe

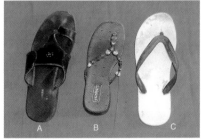

Fig. 10.2: Commonlly worn footwear (chappals) in India

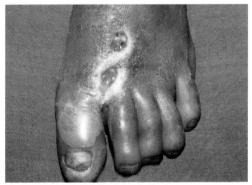

Fig. 10.5: Injury on dorsum of the foot caused due to footwear such as A, B and C

Objects Inside the Shoes

Foreign objects inside the shoes are yet another cause of injuring neuropathic feet. Commonly noticed objects are pebbles, nuts, coins and toys (Fig. 10.6, 10.7), but other objects like ear rings and shoe horn have also been reported. Walking with these foreign bodies tucked inside the shoes, result in pressure necrosis, thus severely damaging the foot. I remember having come across an interesting story in IDF bulletin, narrated by Maria L de Alva, ex-president of IDF. The story was about a Mexican couple who had returned from holidays. The husband who was a diabetic went to work the next day. In the evening when he returned home his wife enquired "Where are my diamond studded earrings?" "I do not know," said the husband, "But I had hidden them in your boots", said the wife. "But certainly not in these boots" said the husband while removing them. And to his great surprise they were in his boots. His foot was swollen and red but not painful, next day he went to his doctor but despite a month's efforts, his leg had to be amputated. It is therefore important to check the footwear before wearing them (Fig. 10.8).

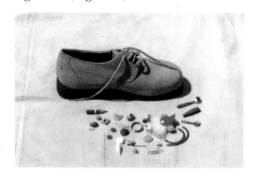

Fig. 10.6: Commonly noticed objects inside the shoe

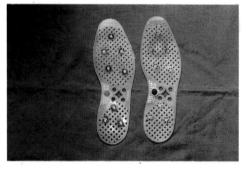

Fig. 10.7: Insoles found in patient's shoes. They were of hard plastic and were stuck with sharp copper buttons (supposed to give a healing touch?)

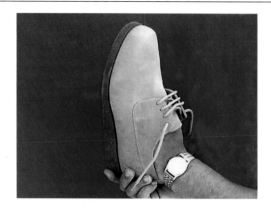

Fig. 10.8: Feel inside the shoe (Fortunately diabetic neuropathy seldom afflicts hands)

Case Study (10.A)

This 60 year old female with type 2 DM of ten years and hypertension of five years duration, presented with swollen great toe right foot since 15 days. History revealed that she had redness and ulceration in the 1st webspace, 20 days back. Prior to this ulceration, she had noticed callosities in both 1st web spaces due to wearing hawaii slippers.

Her general and systemic examinations were normal. Local examination revealed neuropathic feet with a normal ABI, infected and swollen right great toe with ulceration on its lateral aspect and an ulcer in the 1st webspace. There was also a callosity in the left foot 1st webspace (Fig. 10.9 A).

She was hospitalized, switched on to intravenous antibiotics and intensified insulin therapy. Her investigations revealed Hb11.5 gms%, TLC 14100/

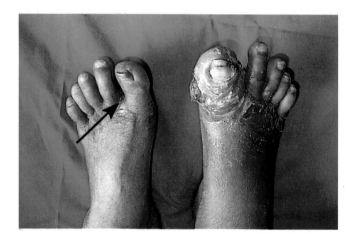

Fig. 10.9A: Showing callosity in 1st web space and grossly infected left great toe as a result of wearing Hawaii chappals.

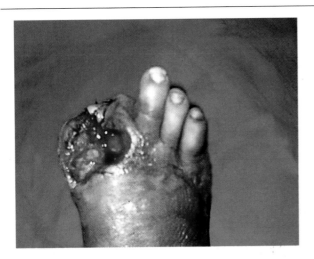

Fig. 10.9B: After debridement and disarticulation at 1st and 2nd MTP joints (open amputation)

cumm, ESR 137 mm/1st hour, S. creatinine 1.5 mg/dL, plasma glucose of 237 mg% and HbA$_{1c}$ 10.7%. She also had evidence of background retinopathy and overt nephropathy; her resting ECG showed sinus tachycardia. Her X-ray of the right foot showed osteomyelitis of both phalanges of the great toe.

A clinical diagnosis of deep seated infection of the right great toe with osteomyelitis and early evidence of soft tissue infection of the 2nd toe was made.

She was subjected to disarticulation of the right foot 1st and 2nd toes at MTP joints and the wound was left open (Fig. 10.9 B). A bacterial swab was sent for culture and sensitivity, which later revealed growth of *staphylococcus aureus*. This wound would eventually require a split skin graft for closure, till then she has been advised strict non weight bearing, wound dressings, insulin, and oral antibiotics.

This severe great toe infection resulted due to ulceration of the 1st webspace callosity which was secondary to friction of the footwear grip. Such infection can readily enter medial compartment and proximally through tendon sheaths to ankle and into the leg, creating a limb threatening situation.

11

Rat Bite

Neuropathic patients should have cats as pets and not dogs
Paul Brand

Patients with neuropathy who sleep on the floor are invariably bitten by house rats who nibble the toes creating ulcerations (Fig.11.1, 11.2). Patients notice the ulcers on waking up in the morning and noticing the blood stained linen. It is interesting how rats selectively bite a neuropathic foot. When a rat strikes at a foot, the normal foot is reflexly withdrawn, whereas the neuropathic foot remains still.

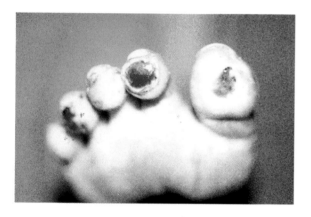
Fig. 11.1: Rat bite ulcers on toes of the right foot

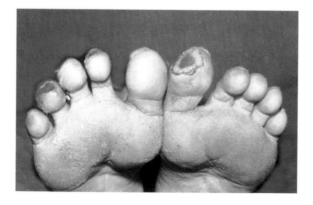
Fig. 11.2: Rat bite ulcers on left 1st toe and right 4th toe

Rat bites have been common in leprosy feet as well. Rats also get attracted by a typical smell of a plantar callus, especially if it is macerated one. Once the rat has successfully nibbled the toes, it often chooses to attack the same person every night and it becomes a recurrent phenomenon. I tell my patients to wear socks at night, use mosquito nets, sleep on the cot and keep the cot in the centre of the room. However, at times rats prove cleverer and on having tasted human flesh, they tend to strike repeatedly.

I know of a lady who was being repeatedly bitten by her house rat. She tried all my tricks but nothing really worked for her. She even tried rat poison cakes. The rat would not touch the cake but religiously strike this lady when she was asleep. Ultimately, I suggested her to wear shoes with a thick outsole. For the last six months, she has been free from rat bites.

Case Study (11.A)

This 56 year old male with a longstanding type 2 diabetes mellitus (DM) and by profession a forest officer, presented with limb threatening infected right foot. There was history of ratbite near first MT head, the patient neglected the ulcer and continued his work in the forest which involved extensive walking.

Local examination revealed swelling over the medial plantar aspect of the forefoot with a ratbite ulcer. There were necrotic ulcers over the medial aspect of 1st MT head and one close to the medial malleolus. The X-ray of the foot revealed destruction of the 1st MTP joint. After initial evaluation, the patient underwent a radical surgical debridement with removal of the 1st metatarsal and the necrotic tissue. Four weeks later, the patient underwent split skin grafting (Fig. 11.3 A to 11.3 D). Although, the wound

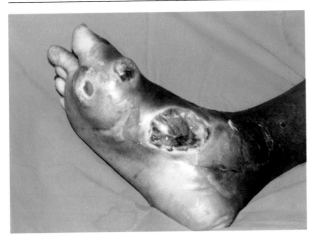

Fig. 11.3A: Advanced infection of the right foot. Note ulcer over 1st MTH. Rats are attracted by a typical smell of macerated plantar callus

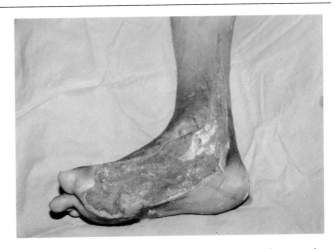

Fig. 11.3B: After the radical debridement and removal of the 1st metatarsal

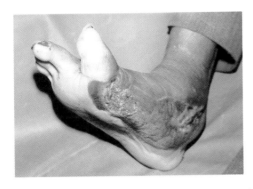

Fig. 11.3C: Defect closed by skin grafting

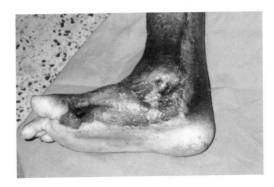

Fig. 11.3D: Six months later

healed the foot was not the same again without the 1st metatarsal. He had to take up a sedentary job and give up his forest officer's post.

So even a trivial ratbite holds in its dark portals such an impending disaster.

12 Thermal Injury

With insensate feet, one can even walk on fire!

In diffuse polyneuropathy in diabetics, both small and large nerve fibers are affected leading to loss of protective sensations of the feet. Rarely they are selectively affected as in painful neuropathy, where selectively small never fiber function is lost like thermal sensation but other sensations like touch and vibration are preserved.

Neuropathic feet are susceptible to thermal injuries due to loss of thermal sensations, which lead to blisters, bullae, excoriation of skin or even full thickness burns. Walking barefoot on hot surfaces, like visiting religious places (religion does not permit wearing shoes), prolonged contact with hot surface during fomentation, silencer pipe of a motor bike, hot water burns during bathing, etc. are some of the causes for thermal trauma (Fig. 12.1 to 12.5). It is not uncommon to see depigmented skin areas, as a result of previous burns in neuropathic feet (Fig. 12.3).

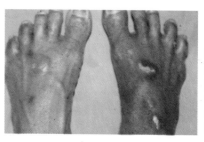

Fig. 12.3: On right dorsum depigmented patches seen signify old thermal injuries, left dorsum showing fresh lesion

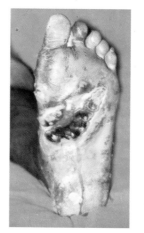

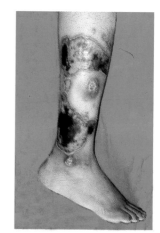

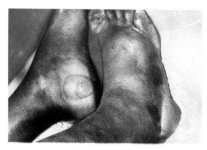

Fig. 12.1: Silencer pipe injury, note bullae over both heels.

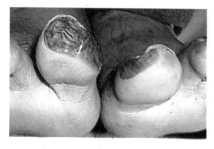

Fig. 12.2: Thermal injury over both great toes. This patient had worn plastic shoes in summer with outside temperature of 46°C

Fig. 12.4: Excoriation of plantar skin after visiting temple barefoot in summer

Fig. 12.5A: Deep burns over right leg after hotwater bag fomentation

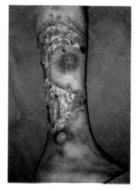

Fig. 12.5B: After debridement

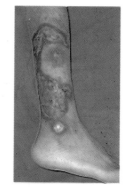

Fig. 12.5C: After skin grafting

INSTRUCTIONS FOR PATIENTS

Diabetic patients with loss of thermal sensation should avoid extremes of both hot and cold temperature. In tropical countries, we do not come across cold injuries, however, literature cites the stories of amputation after prolonged application of cold packs and also frostbite. Patients should be educated to prevent thermal injuries by instructing them to test temperature of water before bathing, visiting temples early morning or late evening, wearing protective footwear when riding pillion on a motor bike or going to hot sandy beaches and should stay away from room heaters or fireplaces during winter.

Case Study (12.A)

This 68 year old female with type 2 DM since 14 years presented with bullae over both feet. History revealed that, she had travelled in a non air-conditioned bus for over four hours during the day time when the outside temperature was 47 degrees celsius. She was wearing hawaii slippers and her feet were touching floor of the bus. She had neuropathic feet and prolonged contact with hot surface led to these bullae. The bullae were deroofed and they healed without scarring (Fig. 12.6 A, 12.6 B). She was advised to wear protective footwear and avoid travel during day time, in summer months.

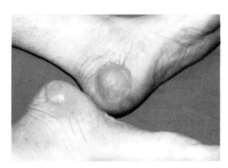

Fig. 12.6A: Bullae over both heels (Thermal injury)

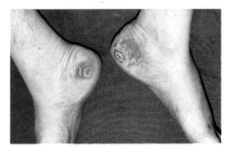

Fig. 12.6B: Wounds healing after deroofing of the bullae

Case Study (12.B)

This 58 year old male with type 2 DM of eight years duration, presented with skin burn on dorsum of right foot. History revealed that he had burning feet syndrome and on the advise of a well wisher, he applied hot sand on his right foot for over 30 minutes. Removal of the sand revealed area of deep burns on the dorsum of foot (Fig. 12.7 A). His wound, although not infected, took eight weeks to heal, and healed with scarring (Fig. 12.7 B). The scar could have been avoided by a split skin graft, had the patient not refused.

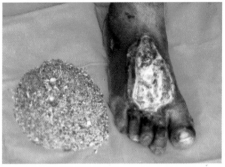

Fig. 12.7A: Deep burns over dorsum of the foot (hot sand fomentation)

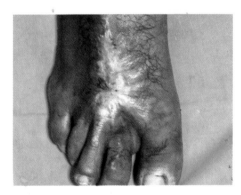

Fig. 12.7B: Wound healed with scarring

Case Study (12.C)

This 63 year old male with type 2 DM of 18 years duration presented with bullous eruption over the lateral margin of left foot. History revealed he was riding pillion on a motorbike, his left foot touching the hot silencer pipe. He was wearing hawaii slippers. He was already diagnosed to have retinopathy both eyes, for which laser was done and nephropathy with early renal insufficiency (S. creatinine 2.4 mg/dl). He had neuropathic feet with normal ABI. He had undergone left foot 5th toe disarticulation, two years ago, because of toe infection (osteomyelitis).

The bulla was deroofed and regularly dressed; the wound healed in two months without any significant scarring (Fig. 12.8 A to 12.8 C).

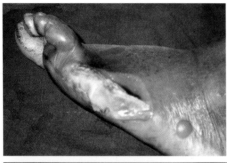

Fig. 12.8A: Bullae after silencer pipe injury

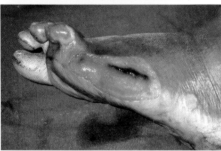

Fig. 12.8B: After deroofing

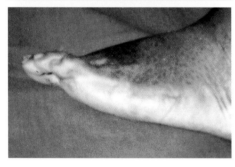

Fig. 12.8C: Wound completely healed

Case Study (12.D)

This 57 year old male with type 2 DM of 12 years duration presented at seven in the evening in our clinic, with bullae over plantar aspect of the left forefoot and tips of toes. Surprisingly though, the right foot escaped. History revealed that he visited a temple four hours ago, barefoot, in a summer month. He had evidence of neuropathy with a normal ABI. The bullae were deroofed and as the ulcerations were superficial, they healed without significant scarring (Fig. 12.9 A, 12.9 B).

As the religion does not permit wearing footwear inside the temples, devotees with DM should be instructed to visit the temples either in the morning or late evening, when the outside temperature is relatively cooler.

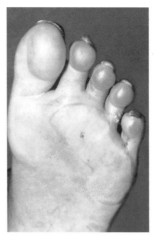
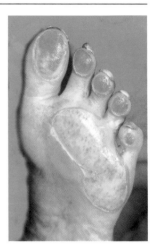

Fig. 12.9A: Bullae over left forefoot and tips of toes after visiting temple barefoot.

Fig. 12.9B: After deroofing, note red floor of the ulcer, suggesting superficial burns

Case Study (12.E)

This 66 year old male with type 2 DM of 11 years duration, presented with a huge bullous eruption over dorsum of the left foot since four hours. He had complaints of burning of feet for which he had applied hot fomentation, using a hot water bag. While the hot water bag was applied to the foot dorsum, he continued to watch the morning news on television. The bag was removed after almost 45 minutes only to reveal a big bulla with a fluid level! He was immediately rushed to our centre. The bulla was deroofed and non adhesive dressing applied (Fig. 12.10 A to 12.10 C). He was sent home and recalled the next morning. However, the patient failed to turn up and returned only after a week. The wound was, surprisingly, covered with necrotic slough. During his week long absence, the wound was being dressed with hot water!

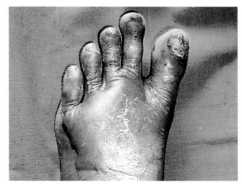

Fig. 12.10A: Bulla over dorsum of the left foot, after hot water bag fomentation

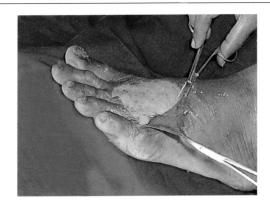

Fig. 12.10B: Bulla being deroofed

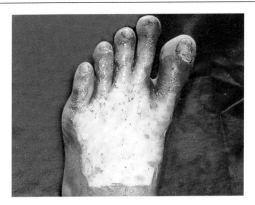

Fig. 12.10C: After deroofing, note pale floor of the ulcer, suggesting deep burns

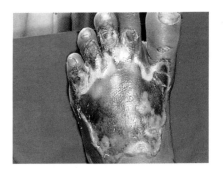

Fig. 12.10D: After 8 days of deroofing, note necrosis of the deeper tissue, indicating deep burns (full thickness)

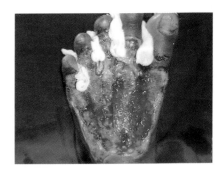

Fig. 12.10E: After debridement

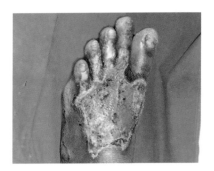

Fig. 12.10F: After skin grafting

He was hospitalized, switched on to intravenous antibiotics and a surgical debridement of the necrotic tissue was carried out. After five days of surgery he was discharged and followed up regularly. Three weeks later, the wound was covered with a split skin graft (Figs 12.10 D to 12.10 F).

Bullous eruptions are superficial (intraepidermal) and usually heal within a few weeks of deroofing, without scarring. In this patient, prolonged hot water fomentation must have led to deep burns (subepidermal), explaining the necrotic slough. Dressings with hot water, at home, must have further worsened the wound.

13 Bullosum Diabeticorum

Bulla is a natural sterile dressing as long as it is intact

Bullae or blisters are superficial fluid filled sacs. Tense blisters or bullae are commonly seen in neuropathic feet. The characteristic history is spontaneous appearance of bullae, usually at the area of friction or secondary to thermal injury, they are often bilateral. Diabetic bullae are of three types depending upon the type of fluid present in them (Fig.13.1 to 13.3), such as:

- Serous
- Hemorrhagic
- Purulent

Common causes of diabetic bullae are (Fig. 13.4 to 13.8) :
- Friction injury, e.g. ill fitting shoes
- Strenuous prolonged walking, e.g. visit to pilgrimage
- Thermal injury, e.g. after hot fomentation, contact with hot surface
- Deep seated abscess in the foot presenting as purulent bulla
- Ischemic ulcer presenting as blister.

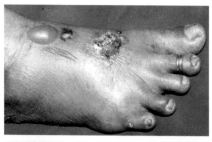

Fig. 13.1: Serous bulla

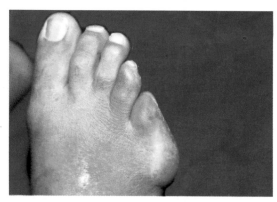

Fig. 13.4: Bulla on the lateral border of the 5th toe due to ill fitting shoe

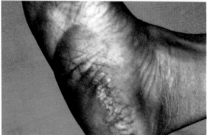

Fig. 13.2: Hemorrhagic bulla

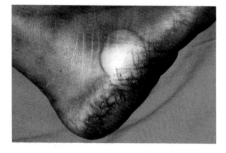

Fig. 13.3: Purulent bulla

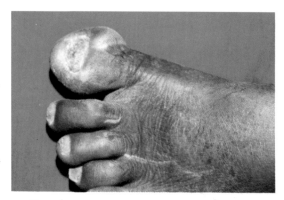

Fig. 13.5: Bulla on the left great toe due to prolonged walking

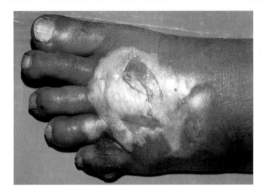

Fig. 13.6: Purulent bulla on the left dorsum, secondary to deep abscess

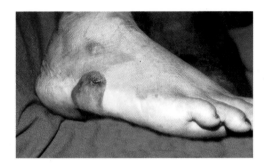

Fig. 13.7A: Hemorrhagic bulla on the lateral border of the right foot due to thermal injury

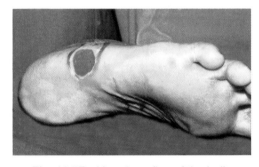

Fig. 13.7B: After deroofing of the bulla

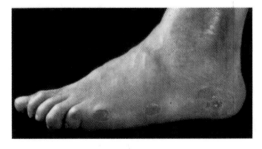

Fig. 13.8: Ischemic ulcers presenting as bullae
(*Courtesy* ME Edmond, AVM Foster, King's College Hospital, London, UK)

MANAGEMENT

If the bullae are small (less than 2 cm), they can be cleaned and covered with a sterile dressing. If large and tense, the bullae should be deroofed with a scalpel or scissors to release the contents before the dressing (Fig.13.9 A to 13.10 B). Aspiration with a syringe is less useful, because the hole may seal and the bullae may become tense again. Patients are tempted to

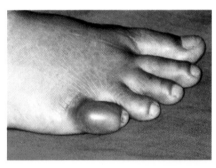

Fig. 13.9A: Bulla on the right 5th toe

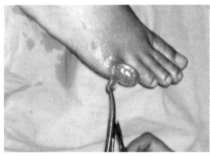

Fig. 13.9B: Bulla being deroofed

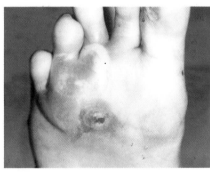

Fig. 13.10A: Bulla secondary to infected plantar ulcer

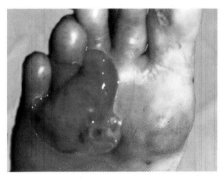

Fig. 13.10B: After deroofing and excision of the ulcer

rupture these bullae at home with unsterile needles, only to convert a sterile bulla into an infected one, which should be discouraged. After deroofing, the lesions heal in a few weeks, usually without scarring. They are often superficial (intra epidermal) explaining the lack of scarring, however few may be deep (subepidermal), and may require prolonged dressings or even debridement and a skin graft. These subepidermal bullae are usually secondary to a prolonged contact with the offending agent. Deroofing of bullae discharging purulent fluid is not enough, they invariably indicate a deep seated infection, and therefore a bold decompression and debridement is often necessary.

14 Lateral Malleolar Bursitis

The price of sitting cross legged

Indians are known for sitting cross legged for long hours at work and during worship. In fact some do not keep a table and chair at the workplace and carry out their business by sitting cross legged. Repeated pressure over lateral malleolar areas lead to formation of bursae on both the feet (Fig.14.1). Similarly Muslims who worship by offering "Namaz" from the age of seven years, five times a day, lifelong, also develop "Namaz" callosities on the left lateral malleolus and dorsolaterally. These callosities develop because of the peculiar position of the left foot during namaz (Fig.14.2).

These bursae over lateral malleoli are pigmented and hypertrophied but are usually harmless in non neuropathic individuals. In diabetics with neuropathy, these bursae get ulcerated due to repeated pressure in absence of pain and often get secondarily infected (Fig. 14.3 A, 14.3 B). Their proximity to heel pad make them vulnerable for creating a limb threatening situation (Fig. 14.4 A, 14.4 B).

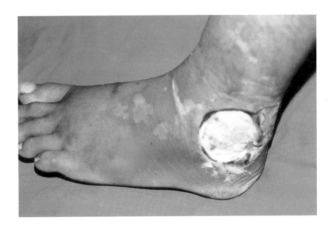

Fig. 14.3A: Ulcerated lateral malleolar bursa with cellulitis

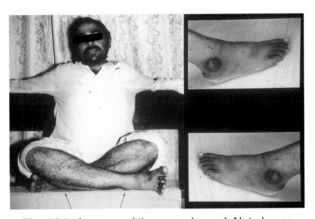

Fig. 14.1: A person sitting cross legged. Note hypertrophied, pigmented bursae over lateral malleoli

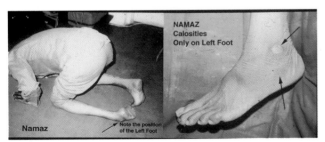

Fig. 14.2: A person offering Namaz, Note position of left leg and callosities on left foot

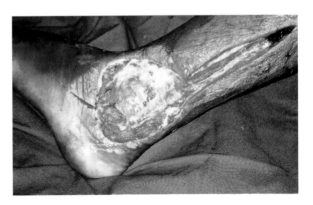

Fig. 14.3B: After debridement

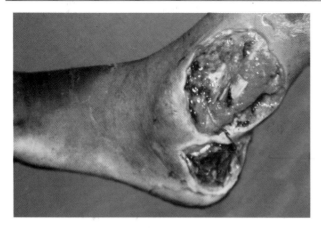

Fig. 14.4A: Infected lateral malleolar bursa, progressing into the heel pad

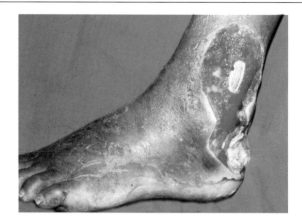

Fig. 14.4B: After radical debridement

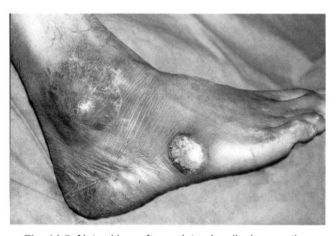

Fig. 14.5: Note skin graft over lateral malleolus, another bursa developed on the lateral border of the foot

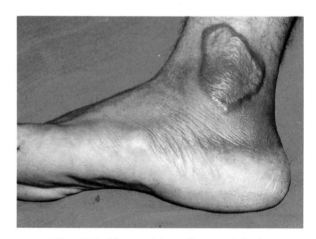

Fig. 14.6: After excision of bursa, defect closed by a skin graft

Infected lateral malleolar bursae need to be surgically excised and the defect closed by split skin grafting (Fig.14.5, 14.6). The patients need to be instructed to avoid sitting in cross legged posture or use a foam cushion with a central hole to suspend the lateral malleoli.

15 Fissures (Cracks)

Fissures result from draught of the plantar skin

It is the abundance of the sweat glands that keeps the plantar skin moist. Sweat glands are controlled by the autonomic nervous system. In DM with autonomic neuropathy, sweating is diminished due to dysfunction of eccrine glands as a result of sympathetic denervation, causing dry skin. Such dry plantar skin (xerosis) can get cracked easily. These cracks are often wide and deep. These are commonly seen in sulci of toes, on the forefoot, and on borders of the heel (Fig. 15.1 to 15.3). Some such cracks and fissures breach the whole skin depth paving way for microorganisms, a threatening forerunner to a deep plantar abscess.

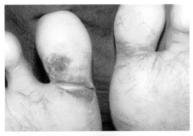

Fig. 15.1: Fissure in sulcus of right great toe

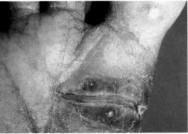

Fig. 15.2: Deep fissure on forefoot

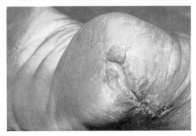

Fig. 15.3: Long and deep fissure on heel

As the changes of autonomic neuropathy are irreversible, patients should be instructed to apply moisturising lotions, oil, or emollient creams. Feet should be thoroughly washed to remove dirt in these fissures. The application of a very thin coat of any vegetable oil to the foot after bathing helps to seal-in the moisture. It is the moisture rather than the oil that keeps the skin pliable and decreases the dryness. It is important that lubricants not be applied in between the toes, because this can cause moisture to accumulate and lead to maceration and infection. If the edges are everted they should be cut by sterile scissors during the clinic visit.

I still remember of a lady who scratched and pulled out the everted skin around these fissures because of intense itching and consequently, her heel got badly infected. She refused any sort of surgical intervention, only to succumb to septicemia.

Trivial looking fissures can be ghastly at times, as evident from various case studies cited elsewhere in this atlas (Case studies 5.A, 5.B, 39.F), where fissures were the initial lesions, which led to the advanced diabetic foot pathology.

Case Study (15.A)

This 40 year old male with type 2 DM of ten years duration, with advanced diabetic retinopathy and overt nephropathy, presented with swelling over left heel and a non healing wound since two weeks. History revealed that he had a deep fissure over the lateral border of the heel, which bled after he tried to pick the skin. His general and systemic examinations were normal. He had neuropathic feet with a normal ABI. His left hindfoot was swollen, with an ulcer on the lateral border of the heel. The ulcer was discharging purulent material, the floor was full of necrotic tissue and slough and the ulcer margins were macerated (Fig. 15.4A). On probing, there was no evidence of osteomyelitis.

He was hospitalized and switched on to IV antibiotics and intensified insulin therapy. His investigations revealed Hb 12.5 gms%, TLC 8600/cu.mm, ESR 89 mm/1st hr, S. creatinine 1 mg/dL, urine albumin was dipstick positive (+++), plasma glucose was 398mg% and HbA$_{1c}$ 10.4%. His retinal examination revealed advanced diabetic retinopathy. His X-ray of the left foot was normal. The duplex Doppler study of the left lower limb arteries revealed a normal triphasic waveform and patent posterior tibial artery. A diagnosis of infected left heel ulcer without osteomyelitis was made. He was subjected to surgical debridement and the slough and necrotic tissues were removed. The deep cavity (Fig. 15.4 B) after removal of necrotic tissue, filled-up in 4 weeks with granulation tissue (Fig. 15.4 C). This wound should heal by epithelization.

Heel pad infections are notorious for non-healing, the prognosis worsens if the infection is deep seated and is worst if there is osteomyelitis of the calcaneus.

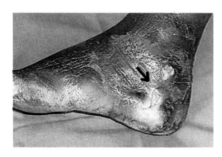

Fig. 15.4A: Infected fissure left heel with maceration of surrounding skin

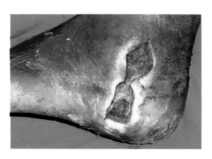

Fig. 15.4B: After debridement, note deep cavity

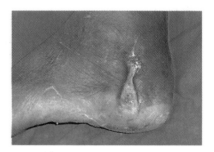

Fig. 15.4C: Healing wound

16 Intrinsic Minus Foot

Small muscle loss leads to large structural defect

Peripheral diabetic neuropathy involves all the three components of the peripheral nervous system leading to autonomic, motor, and sensory neuropathies. Intrinsic minus foot occurs secondary to motor neuropathy. The small intrinsic musculature of the foot begins to atrophy due to loss of motor innervation of small muscles like lumbricals and interossei.

Lumbricals

There are four lumbricals which arise from the tendons of the flexor digitorum longus to get inserted into the base of the proximal phalanges. Their action is to adduct the lateral four toes towards the great toe.

Interossei

There are three plantar interossei which lie below the metatarsals and four dorsal interossei which arise from metatarsals and lie between them. Plantar interossei adduct the lateral three toes towards second toe, whereas the dorsal interossei abduct them from midline of the second toe. They also assist in flexing the metatarsophalangeal joints and extending the interphalangeal joints.

Loss of function and contractures of interossei predispose to ulcers on dorsum of the digits. It also increases the pressure underneath the MT heads. The peroneal nerve involvement can produce unilateral or bilateral foot drop, which is often unrecognized until such time it has developed a fixed equinus deformity. Motor neuropathy leads to changes in the foot structure and joint patterns. The intrinsic minus foot has been ascribed to atrophy of the intrinsic muscles which control the position of the proximal phalanges on the metatarsals. It leads to contracted digits, claw toes, hammer toes, crowding of toes, and exaggeration of bunions (Figs 16.1 to 16.2B). The gait also becomes unstable.

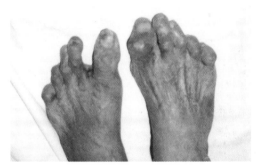

Fig. 16.1: Instrinsic minus feet, note muscle atrophy, clawing of toes

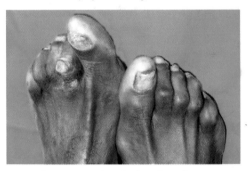

Fig. 16.2A: Instrinsic minus feet, note bunion on the 2nd toe left

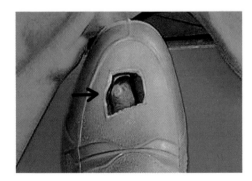

Fig. 16.2B: The patient created a window in the uppers of his shoe to prevent ulceration of bunion (seen through window). Innovative patient!

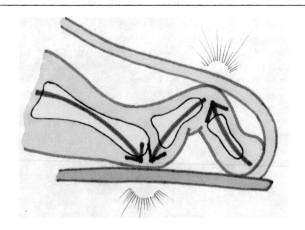

Fig. 16.3: Toe deformities increase friction with the uppers of shoe, increasing risk of ulceration on the dorsum of toes

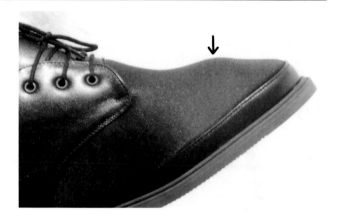

Fig. 16.4: Shoe with elastic uppers to accommodate toe deformities, thus reducing friction

The intrinsic minus foot thus leads to high risk areas for foot ulcerations on the tips of toes, underneath MT heads, and dorsum of the IP joints (Fig. 16.3). Footwear with a high toe box and extra depth help to accommodate such toe deformities and prevent friction injuries. Elastic uppers being stretchable are also used in shoes, to accommodate the toe deformities (Fig. 16.4).

17 Deformities

Deformities are surrogate markers of raised plantar pressure
Cavanagh, Ulbrecht, Caputo

Bony deformities increase the risk of foot ulceration several folds in a neuropathic foot. They result as a consequence of sensory and motor neuropathy. Deformities lead to bony prominences, areas of high localized pressure, and the total weight bearing area of the foot is reduced. The overlying or underlying skin is subjected to a high mechanical pressure. In neuropathic foot, the response to high pressure is hyperkeratosis and callus formation with eventual ulceration, whereas in neuroischemic foot, pressure leads to direct tissue damage and ulceration. Even callus requires a good blood supply to grow, thus explaining its flourishing growth in neuropathic foot as compared to neuroischemic foot. Deformities should be recognized early and accommodated in extra depth shoes with a high toe box and a soft insole, before any ulceration occurs. Common deformities seen in diabetics are discussed below.

DEFORMITIES OF TOES

Hallux Valgus

It is a deformity of the great toe at the metatarso-phalangeal (MTP) joint. The hallux deviates laterally (adduction) in relation to the first metatarsal head and shaft. A bony prominence, exostosis, appears over the head of metatarsal (MT) medially (Figs 17.1 to 17.2B). Repeated friction (ill fitting shoe) can result in a bursa, which eventually ulcerates facilitating spread of infection in MTP joint and medial compartment of foot. Hallux valgus deformity can also occur after the disarticulation of the second toe (Fig. 17.22). If a toe spacer is not used, the great toe deviates laterally due to lack of support of the second toe.

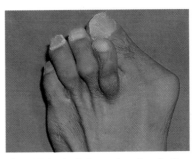

Fig. 17.1: Left foot showing hallux valgus, crowding of toes prominent tendons due to small muscle atrophy

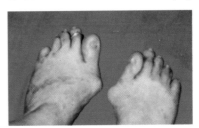

Fig. 17.2A: Showing bilateral hallux valgus

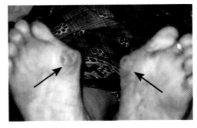

Fig. 17.2B: Callus on 1st MT heads

Hallux Rigidus

It is really not a deformity but dysfunction of the great toe. It leads to diminished mobility of the first MTP joint with diminished ability to dorsiflex the great toe. It results because of limited joint mobility (LJM) due to nonenzymatic glycosylation of proteins. The risk of ulceration is on the ball of the great toe.

Hallux Varus

Medial deviation of the hallux is hallux varus. It is relatively rare and is often seen in patients with neuro-arthropathy of MTP joint (Fig. 17.3).

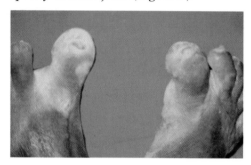

Fig. 17.3: Bilateral hallux varus

Cock-Up Deformity

It is seen in the great toe. The IP joint is flexed, and the MTP joint is extended (Fig. 17.4). The deformity is caused by an imbalance between flexor and extensor muscles of the great toe. The risk of ulceration is increased on the dorsum of the IP joint and plantar surface (ball) of the great toe.

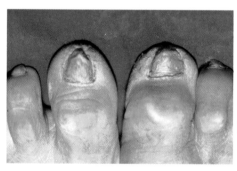

Fig. 17.4: Cock-up deformity of both great toes

Claw Toes

Atrophy of small muscle of foot due to motor neuropathy (Intrinsic minus foot) results in clawed toes. There is a flexion deformity at the IP joint and dorsiflexion of MTP joint. Risk of ulceration is increased on dorsum and tips of the toes (Fig. 17.5).

Hammer Toe

The loss of balancing lumbrical function results in hammer toe. MTP joint of the toe is extended, and the

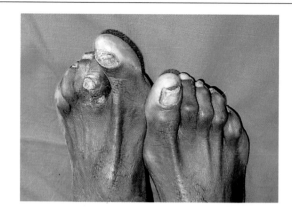

Fig. 17.5: Clawed toes with bunion 2nd left toe

proximal IP joint is flexed. It may occur in one or several toes of the same foot. The risk areas for ulceration are dorsum of toes at the proximal IP joint and tips of the toes (Fig. 17.6).

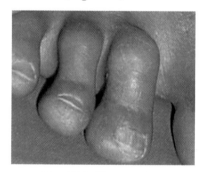

Fig. 17.6: Hammer toes

Mallet Toe

It involves the distal IP joint, the distal phalanx is flexed on the proximal phalanx. It is usually seen in 2nd toe (Fig. 17.7), which is often the longest ray of the foot but can also involve other toes of the same foot. No mallet deformity exists with hallux.

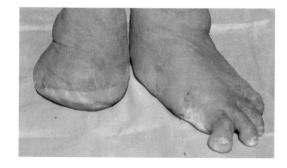

Fig. 17.7: Mallet toe left 2nd toe, also note varus deformity of the 2nd toe due to loss of support of the great toe, Right transmetatarsal amputation

Varus Deformities of the Toes

The third, fourth, and fifth toes deviate medially, which may cause nails to gouge adjacent toes, producing ulcers. Crowding of toes results in increased risk of interdigital infection due to poor hygiene and overlapping of toes can cause skin friction of toe on toe (Figs 17.8A and B).

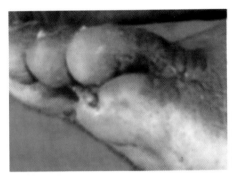

Fig. 17.8A: Varus deformities of toes (left) with overriding 4th toe

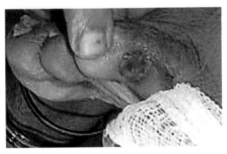

Fig. 17.8B: Ulcer on the 4th toe due to friction of toe on toe

Bunion

It is an exostosis seen commonly over the dorsum of toes on the IP joints. It results because of combination of claw toes and tight footwear (Fig. 17.9). Ulceration at this site can rapidly cause septic arthritis of IP joint.

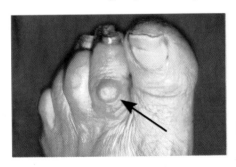

Fig. 17.9: Bunion left 2nd toe

Tailor's Bunion (Bunionette)

It is characterized by a prominence of lateral eminence of 5th MT head. Pressure over lateral condyle of 5th MT head leads to chronic irritation of the overlying bursa. The position of a tailor sitting in a "crosslegged position" apparently has given rise to the term "tailor's bunion". It is analogus to the medial eminence of the 1st MT head in a hallux valgus deformity. The loss of abduction function of dorsal interossei causes toes to become crowded on the axis of the 2nd toe, accentuating the angular prominence of the 5th MTP joint (Fig. 17.10). Ulceration at this site can spread into MTP joint of the fifth toe and lateral plantar compartment.

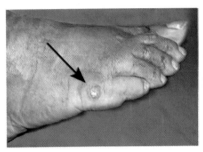

Fig. 17.10: Bunionette

DEFORMITIES OF FOOT

Pes Cavus

Medial longitudinal arch of the foot is formed posteriorly by calcaneus and anteriorly by the first three metatarsal heads. Exaggeration of this arch is called as pes cavus (Figs 17.11 and 17.12). It leads to prominent head of the first metatarsal and the risk of ulceration is increased underneath its head.

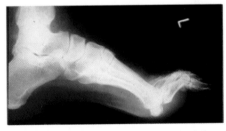

Fig. 17.11: Radiograph showing pes cavus deformity, note thinned out subcutaneous tissue underneath 1st MT head, increasing risk of ulceration

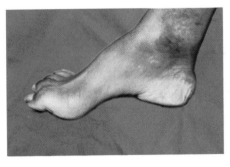

Fig. 17.12: Pes cavus deformity of right foot

Pes Planus

Pes planus is also referred to as a flat foot. Normally, the medial arch of foot prevents medial portion of mid foot from ground contact, during midstance position. In pes planus, medial arch is flattened and the area at risk is medial portion of the mid foot. Unilateral, acquired pes planus deformity can be an early feature of the Charcot foot (Fig. 17.14). Pes planus (flat foot) is also seen in normal individuals, it assumes importance in diabetic individuals with neuropathy (Fig. 17.13).

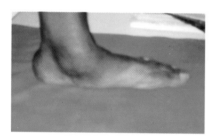

Fig. 17.13: Flat foot (left)

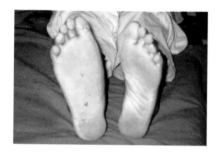

Fig. 17.14: Pes planus due to Charcot foot right with loss of medial arch, left foot normal

Medial Convexity of Foot

This deformity is seen in Charcot foot. It results from tarso-metatarsal dislocation or from displacement of talonavicular joint. The risk of ulceration is increased at medial side of the foot at the convexity or underneath the convexity (Fig. 17.15).

Rocker Bottom Deformity

It is a characteristic deformity secondary to Charcot joint due to collapse of medial arch of foot (Fig. 17.16). It occurs as a result of displacement and subluxation of the tarsus downwards because of neuro-arthropathy. Such a foot rocks on the midfoot. Normally, mid foot ulceration is rare, however this

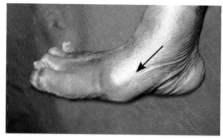

Fig. 17.15: Medial convexity right foot (medial view)

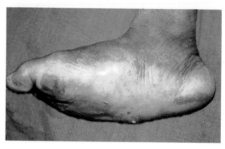

Fig. 17.16: Rocker bottom deformity of Charcot foot

deformity increases the risk several times. Managing midfoot ulceration is extremely difficult (see also Charcot foot). Prevention of ulceration can be achieved by minimum weight bearing and use of extra depth footwear and molded insoles.

Ankle Deformities

They are invariably seen with severe neuro-arthropathy due to Charcot foot. It leads to ankle valgus deformity (Fig. 17.17) or a flail ankle. Once the ankle joint is grossly damaged as in flail ankle (Fig. 17.18), stability of foot is lost, making walking almost impossible. Such destructed and deformed ankle often ends in BK amputation.

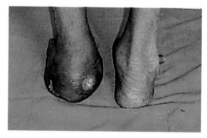

Fig. 17.17: Ankle valgus deformity left (Charcot foot)

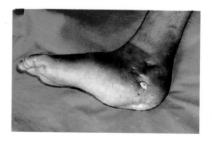

Fig. 17.18: Flail ankle due to Charcot foot

DEFORMITIES AFTER FOOT SURGERY

Radical debridement foot surgeries often involve resection of muscles, tendons, bones and even nerves, which leads to imbalance of muscles resulting in toe and foot deformities.

Toe Deformities

Figure 17.19 shows toe deformities in the right foot, after debridement surgery (scar seen on the dorsum). Figure 17.20 shows extension of the great toe after removal of 1st metatarsal (Hallux extensus).

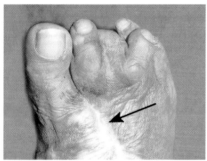

Fig. 17.19: Toe deformities post debridement (scar seen)

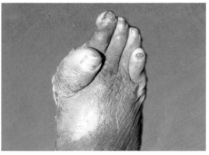

Fig. 17.20: Hallux extensus after removal of 1st metatarsal

Crablike Deformity

This deformity is seen after amputation of the middle toes. The lack of support of adjacent toes leads to hallux valgus deformity of the great toe and varus deformities of remaining toes both trying to reach each other giving the appearance of the pincers of a crab (Figs 17.21 and 17.22).

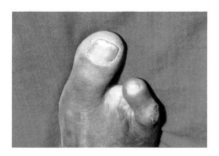

Fig. 17.21: Crablike deformity

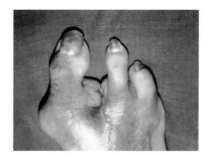

Fig. 17.22: Hallux valgus after removal of 2nd and 3rd toes right foot

Varus Deformity of the Foot

Foot is inverted and usually results secondary to extensive debridement surgery. Figure 17.23A shows such a varus deformity of the foot in a patient who continued to walk on the lateral border of the foot, causing ulceration (Fig. 17.23 B).

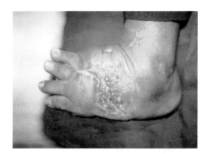

Fig. 17.23A: Varus deformity of the foot

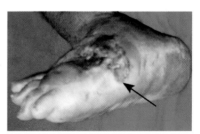

Fig. 17.23B: Leading to ulcer on lateral border of the foot

For most of the toe deformities preventive footwear, which have extra depth, soft insoles, and a tall toe box are essential to accommodate the deformities and prevent pressure injuries. Footwear with flexible elastic uppers accommodate dorsal deformities and prevent friction injuries. The patients with foot deformities often need customized footwear with molded insoles.

18 Limited Joint Mobility (LJM)

Foot is no more supple and resilient

Limited joint mobility was originally described in type 1 DM and was also referred to as diabetic cheiropathy. It consists of two major components, limitation of mobility, primarily of small joints of hands with thickening and stiffness of skin (pseudoscleroderma). It is bilateral, symmetric and painless. It can be demonstrated as an inability to oppose fingertips and palmar surfaces of the fingers of the opposite hands (Prayer Sign) (Figs 18.1 and 18.2). Diabetic cheiropathy is a clinical marker of poorly managed type 1 DM and is invariably associated with advanced microangiopathic complications. The prevalence of this condition has markedly diminished in last two decades with a better understanding of the management of type 1 DM and emphasis on a tight glycemic control with multiple injections of insulin.

Recently the syndrome of limited joint mobility (LJM) has been recognized as an important contributor to abnormal mechanics and foot pressures in diabetic foot. However, the risk of foot ulceration increases only if LJM is associated with sensory neuropathy. In LJM, the joints are not directly involved. Nonenzymatic glycosylation (NEG) of proteins and accompaniment of persistent hyperglycemia, leads to abnormalities in periarticular collagen tissues.

CLINICAL DIAGNOSIS

The important movements of the joints of foot are, dorsiflexion and plantar flexion (small joints of foot as well as ankle), while those of the subtalar joint are inversion and eversion.

Hallux Rigidus

LJM leads to a rigid great toe. Dorsiflexion of great toe is limited thus increasing the pressure on plantar skin of the IP joint and increasing the risk of ulceration on ball of the great toe, especially during the toe-off phase of gait cycle (Fig. 18.3). Hallux rigidus can be demonstrated by asking the patient to dorsiflex the

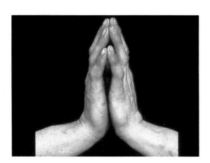

Fig. 18.1: Prayer sign (diabetic cheiropathy), note inability to oppose palmar surfaces of fingers

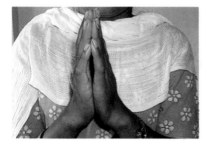

Fig. 18.2: Diabetic cheiropathy in a 20 years old girl with poorly managed Type 1 diabetes on once a day lente insulin

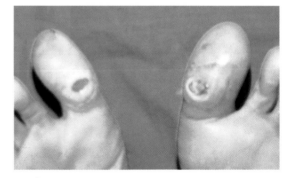

Fig. 18.3: Bilateral hallux ulcers, as a result of hallux rigidus

great toe. The angle between ground and the great toe should be 15° (Fig. 18.4).

Testing the Ankle Joint

Ask the patient to stand on heel and dorsiflex the forefoot. Normal angle between the ground and the foot should be 15° (Fig. 18.5). Next ask the patient to stand on forefoot with heel up. Normal angle between the ground and the heel (heel up position) should be 45° (Fig. 18.6).

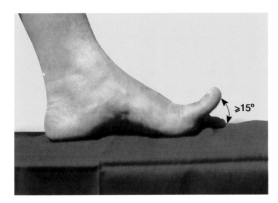

Fig. 18.4: Testing for hallux rigidus, note the normal angle

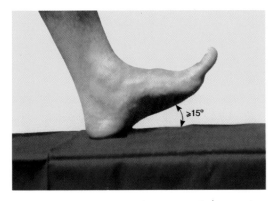

Fig. 18.5: Testing the ankle joint, note the normal angle

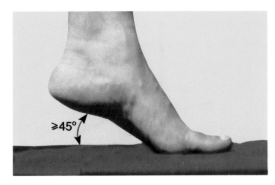

Fig. 18.6: Heel up position, note the normal angle

Testing the Subtalar Joint

Hold the lower leg, move the calcaneus medially and laterally and ask the patient to carry out inversion and eversion respectively.

Limited Mobility of Plantar Skin and Soft Tissues

The flexibility and suppleness of plantar tissue make walking, jumping, turning and dancing look so easy.

While the foot is standing on the ground, it is rather like an arch. Posterior pillar of the arch is calcaneus and anterior pillar is made up of all the bones of the forefoot. This bony arch of the foot is stabilized by soft tissues like ligaments and plantar aponeurosis. These tissues are soft and springy and work like a bowstring. When this bowstring is tightened the two pillars move closer and the arch becomes higher and when the bowstring relaxes the arch becomes relatively flat. NEG of proteins not only affects the periarticular collagen fibers but also collagen and elastic tissue, keratin of plantar skin and soft tissues. Normally foot is supple and resilient and thus while walking pressure is constantly transmitted from one to another area. LJM and limited mobility of skin and soft tissues make the foot rigid and nonelastic, thus increasing the pressure and risk of foot ulceration especially in presence of sensory neuropathy.

Treatment

There is no drug treatment for the rigid and contracted foot, secondary to LJM. However, now there is preliminary evidence that mobilization exercises may be effective in increasing the range of motion of joints of the foot (Fig. 18.7) and perhaps also in reducing

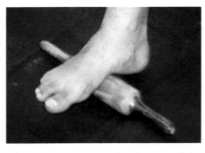

Fig. 18.7: Exercising with a rolling pin, to increase range of motion at joints (A practice to use glass bottle could be dangerous)

plantar pressure during walking. The mobilization exercises are stretching the toes in flexion and extension, foot in inversion and eversion, forefoot in adduction and abduction, and ankle in dorsiflexion and plantar flexion.

19 Plantar Callus

We should not be callous towards a Callus

Body's natural protective response to any palmar or plantar skin irritation, is hyperkeratosis. Plantar skin of farmers or tribals who walk at least 10 miles (15 k.m.) a day, barefoot, on all sorts of uneven surfaces develop thick hyperkeratinized plantar skin. Similarly, we experience overnight thickening and hyperkeratoses on heads of metacarpals in our hands, if we perform strenuous and unaccustomed exercises like gardening. In the presence of normal sensations such hyperkeratosis is a protective mechanism.

Plantar callus on the other hand is a localized hyperkeratosis found at the site of elevated plantar pressures and chronic friction in the insensitive foot. Callus grows to a greater extent in a neuropathic foot, than in a neuroischemic foot, as even the growth of a callus requires a good blood supply. Although for its growth vascularity is essential, callus by itself is avascular. The growth of callus further elevates the already elevated plantar pressure. The intervening soft tissue, between the callus and the bony prominence, gets damaged with every loading step (walking). Callus is commonly seen in the forefoot especially on its medial margin, on ball of the great toe, underneath the metatarsal heads, tips of the lesser toes, rarely in mid foot and hindfoot. It grows around the rim of a plantar ulcer like a halo and also at the site of increased plantar pressure after partial foot amputation due to altered biomechanics (Figs 19.1 to 19.8).

Sites of Plantar Callus

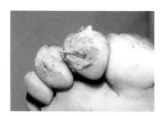

Fig. 19.1: Tips of the lesser toes

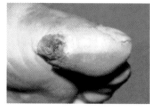

Fig. 19.2: Medial margin of the great toe

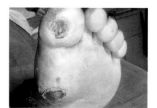

Fig. 19.3: Ball of the great toe and 1st MT head

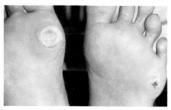

Fig. 19.4: Right 1st MT head, left 5th MT head

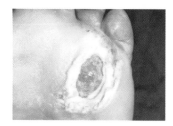

Fig. 19.5: (Like a halo) Around the ulcer rim

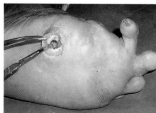

Fig. 19.6: Mid foot

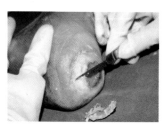

Fig. 19.7: Heel

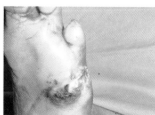

Fig. 19.8: After toe amputations

Removal of Callus

The precursor of plantar ulcer is the development of a callus. If left untreated, the underlying soft tissue gets damaged and breaks down eventually. In fact, studies have shown that removal of callus leads to reduction in plantar pressure by an average of 29%. Fissuring and cracking in the callus leads to central excavation and increased risk of infection (Fig. 19.12). Hematoma in the callus is an ominous sign and must be taken as seriously as an ulcer (Figs 19.13A and B). It is therefore strongly recommended that callus be looked for and that appropriate measures be taken to prevent, limit, and remove it.

Removal of Callus

The callus should be removed with a scalpel, ensuring

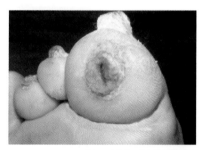

Fig. 19.9A: Thick growth on the ball of great toe

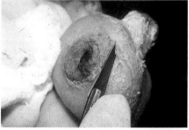

Fig. 19.9B: Removal using a scalpel

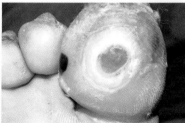

Fig. 19.9C: Preexisting ulcer seen after callus removal

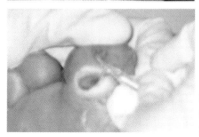

Fig. 19.10: Removal of callus around the rim of plantar ulcer

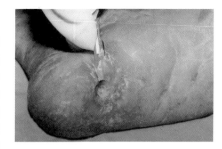

Fig. 19.11A: Around heel ulcer rim

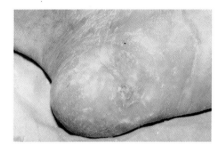

Fig. 19.11B: Healing ulcer after callus removal and off-loading

that the fingers of the other hand maintain a good skin tension (Fig.19.9A to 19.11B). The removal should be just enough deep, as to avoid bleeding. If the callus is thick, do not try to cut it one piece. Sharp debridement should only be performed by experts, as uneven removal can lead to focal points of high pressures and can make future callus removal difficult. Speckles of blood or a deeper layer of whitish, macerated, moist tissue found under the surface of the callus indicate that the foot is close to ulceration (Fig. 19.14). Removal of callus often reveals a preexisting plantar ulcer which needs to be attended to immediately (Fig. 19.9 C).

The callus should not be allowed to grow too thick and hence it should be removed periodically (monthly visit). If it reforms rapidly, it indicates that there are high pressures, acting on the plantar surface of the foot, which need redistribution with a proper footwear

Bad signs of prognosis

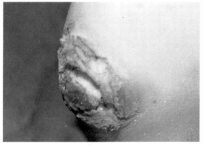

Fig. 19.12: Excessive growth with cracking-up of the callus

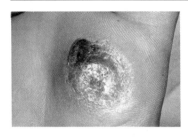

Fig. 19.13A: Hemorrhage in the callus

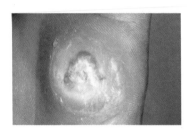

Fig. 19.13B: Speckles of blood after removal of the callus

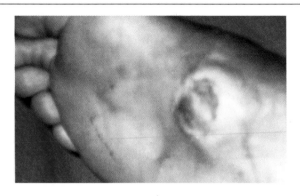

Fig. 19.14: (White) Macerated callus

and insoles. One measure to know how effective the footwear is, is its ability to prevent callus.

Instruction for Patients

- Never cut a callus or use corn removers
- However contribute to limiting callus, by daily self care and filing the callus with a pumice-stone.

20 Charcot Foot

In extreme cases, the foot is like a bag of loose bones

The Charcot foot or neuro-arthropathy is defined as a relatively painless, progressive, and destructive arthropathy in a single or multiple joints, due to underlying neuropathy. Although, the Charcot foot was originally described in tertiary syphilis, it is also seen in many other conditions like syringomyelia, leprosy, and diabetes mellitus. I have seen garden varieties of the Charcot feet in leprosy patients (see chapter 22 on lessons from leprosy foot {Fig. 22.1}). However, with the prevalence of leprosy being reduced globally with a simultaneous increase in the prevalence of diabetes mellitus, diabetic neuropathy is presently the commonest cause of the Charcot foot.

PATHOGENESIS

Multiple factors appear to contribute to the development of the Charcot foot. A peripheral neuropathy with loss of protective sensation, an autonomic neuropathy with increased blood flow to the bone, and mechanical trauma, have emerged as the most important determinants. Basically, there is increased an osteoclastic (bone resorption) activity over an osteoblastic (bone deposition) activity. The autonomic neuropathy leads to an arterial dilatation (sympathetic denervation) and arteriovenous shunting, increasing blood flow which in turn causes bone resorption. The loss of protective pain sensation and presence of uninterrupted physical activity finally make these osteopenic bones susceptible to stress fractures, bone destruction, and collapse of the foot architecture.

JOINT INVOLVEMENT

Although, any joint of the foot can be involved, the most frequent location of neuro-arthropathy is the tarsal-metatarsal region, followed by metatarso-phalangeal joint, the ankle, subtalar, and then the interphalangeal joints. Radiologically, metatarsals show an atrophy or osteolysis of bone, often described as a "sucked candy" and "mortar and pestle" appearance of the MTP or IP joint. An X-ray foot can also reveal fragmentation, fracture, new bone formation, subluxation and dislocation of the joints (Figs 20.1 to 20.4).

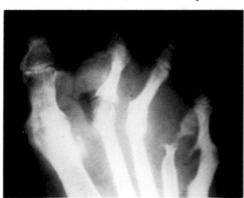

Fig. 20.1: Radiograph showing osteolytic destruction of MTP joints

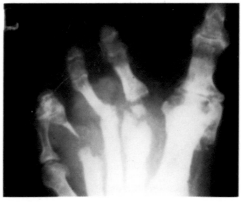

Fig. 20.2: Radiograph showing osteolytic destruction of MTP joints with fragmentation 2nd MTP joint, pencil like narrowing of 4th toe phalanx.

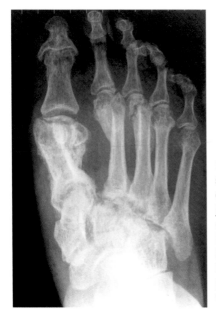

Fig. 20.3: Radiograph showing involvement of tarsometatarsal joints with lateral displacement of MT bases, note pathological fracture of 3rd MT head and "mortar-pestle" appearance of the 1st IP joint

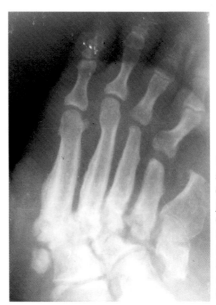

Fig. 20.4: Radiograph showing involvement of tarsometatarsal joints with lateral displacement of MT bases, bone fragmentation, tapering of 2nd and 3rd MT shafts resembling a "sucked candy" appearance

CLINICAL PRESENTATION

The clinical presentation of Charcot foot can be divided into three phases:
- Acute onset
- Bony destruction/deformity
- Stabilization

Acute Onset

Classically, the Charcot foot at its acute onset is hot, erythematous, and swollen with bounding pulses and prominent veins (Figs 20.5 to 20.7). Usually the pain or discomfort is minimal due to underlying neuropathy. A history of recent injury will often precedes onset of the swelling. It is important to differentiate the acute stage of Charcot foot from cellulitis, as both have a red, hot, and swollen foot. Few differentiating features are: cellutitis is more likely in the presence of an ulcer which may show signs of infection, it is usually associated with fever, raised total leukocyte counts, and raised erythrocyte sedimentation rate. An X-ray of the foot may be normal in the acute stage of Charcot. However, technetium di-phosphonate bone scan may detect early bone damage.

Management

Prevention of further trauma is the primary goal in treating the acute phase of Charcot foot. Rest to the swollen foot helps the acute process to subside and allows conversion to a reparative, quiescent stage. This imperative requires an initial period of non-weight bearing to eliminate all stress from the injured foot.

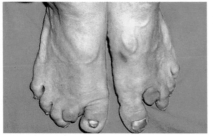

Fig. 20.5: Prominent veins because of arteriovenous shunting (Autonomic neuropathy)

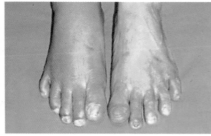

Fig. 20.6: Acute stage of Charcot foot right note redness and swelling

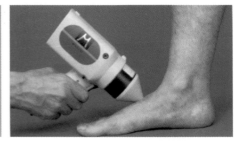

Fig. 20.7: Infrared thermometer to measure skin temperature
(Courtesy ME Edmonds and A V M Foster, King's College Hospital, London, UK)

Total bed rest is the best option, but is not acceptable one in most of the cases. Complete off-loading, using crutches or a wheel chair, will result in fairly rapid reduction in the swelling. After a month, a total contact cast is applied and the patient is mobilized for brief periods. Such a treatment, if given early, should help prevent the second phase, which is that of bone destruction. Once the acute stage subsides, a gradual mobilization may be tried. The patient should be instructed to use his feet to a minimum possible, to prevent a recurrence.

Bone Destruction/Deformity

Clinically the foot is swollen, warm and the medial arch of the foot is usually collapsed. An X-ray reveals fragmentation, fracture, new bone formation, subluxation, and dislocation. These changes develop very rapidly, within a few weeks of the onset. Classical deformities of the Charcot foot are a rockerbottom foot, a medial convexity and ankle deformities (Figs 20.8 to 20.10B). Involvement of tarso-metatarsal joints leads to altered shape of the foot. The mid foot appears broad and the medial arch is collapsed. Involvement of MTP and IP joint lead to deformities of the toes and the ankle joint involvement leads to a swollen hindfoot and deformities of the ankle (Figs 20.11A to 20.13).

Management

The aim of the treatment is immobilization until there is no longer evidence of continuing bone destruction on radiological examination. The medial arch collapse leads to an increased risk of mid foot ulceration, which may become infected and lead to osteomyelitis. The

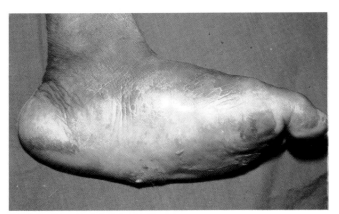

Fig. 20.8: Rocker bottom deformity

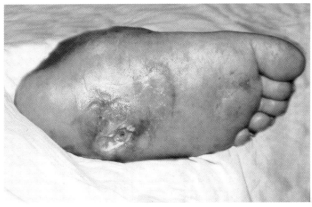

Fig. 20.9: Midfoot ulceration in left Charcot foot

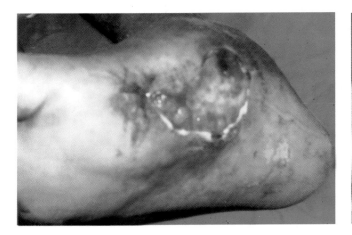

Fig. 20.10A: Medial convexity right Charcot foot with infected ulcer

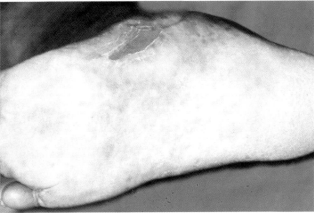

Fig. 20.10B: After control of infection wound closed with a skin graft

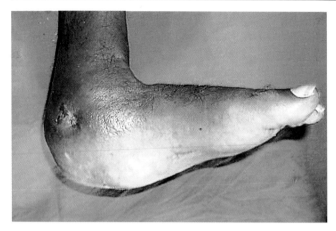

Fig. 20.11A: Ankle deformity of left Charcot foot, medial view, see radiograph of the same patient (Fig. 20.11B)

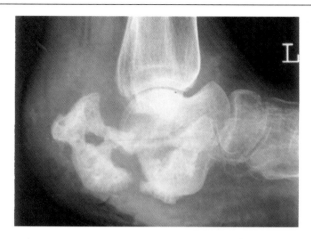

Fig. 20.11B: Radiograph showing collapse of talonavicular, naviculo- cuneiform and calcaneocuboid joints with osteolytic destruction of calcaneus

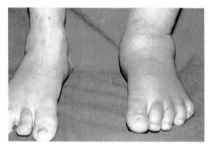

Fig. 20.12A: Front view showing flail ankle left

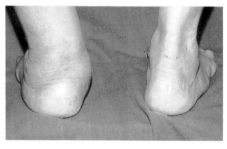

Fig. 20.12B: View from behind showing flail ankle left

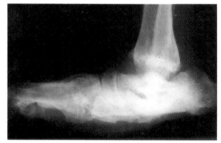

Fig. 20.13: Radiograph lateral view showing collapse of talonavicular and calcaneo-cuboid joints

management of mid foot ulcer without osteomyelitis is removal of callus, control of infection, and strict off-loading (Figs 20.14A to 20.14C). While the management of mid foot ulceration with osteomyelitis (Fig. 20.15) is extremely difficult and can often lead to a major amputation. The treatment is prolonged I/V antibiotics, surgical debridement, and strict off-loading.

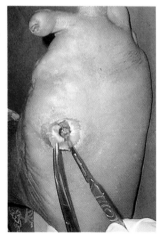

Fig. 20.14A: Mid foot ulcer, callus being removed

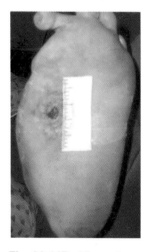

Fig. 20.14B: After callus removal

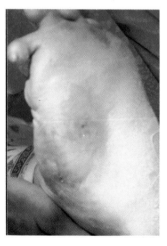

Fig. 20.14C: Healing mid foot ulcer, after off-loading

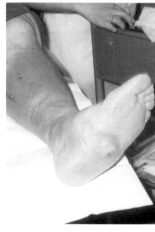

Fig. 20.15: Infected mid foot ulcer with cellulitis left leg

Non-weight bearing is the key for conversion of phase of bone destruction to a stage of stabilization. The principles of non-weight bearing are similar to those described in the management of the acute stage.

Stabilization

The foot is no longer red or swollen. From several weeks of immobilization, the patients can be gradually weaned off to some degree of mobilization. Molded insoles alongwith extra depth and a wide footwear should be advocated. Too rapid a mobilization can be dangerous, resulting in further bone destruction. Regular shaving of the callus at the site of raised pressure can prevent mid foot ulceration.

PROGNOSIS

It depends mainly on the amount of destruction that has taken place. This is directly as a result of the amount of trauma or weight bearing sustained by the joint whilst in the stage of bone destruction. If the Charcot foot is diagnosed early and a strict non-weight bearing is instituted, there will be an arrest of the joint destruction and early conversion to the stage of stabilization. There will be less morbidity and a greater likelihood of stable fusion or reconstruction taking place.

However, if the diagnosis is delayed with continued weight bearing during the stages of acute onset or bone destruction, which is often the case, the prognosis is poor. The bone destruction continues, healing is delayed, significant deformities develop with attendant instability, abnormal weight bearing surfaces, ulceration and infection. The most serious complication of the Charcot foot is instability of the hindfoot and ankle joint. This can lead to flail ankle on which it is impossible to walk. The foot in the worst cases is reduced to a bag of loose bones; culminating in a leg amputation.

21 Local Gigantism

Gulliver among Lilliputians

Non-inflammatory enlargement of a toe or toes secondary to recurrent neuropathic ulcerations is called local gigantism (Figs 21.1 to 21.4). The toe is almost double the original size and should not be confused with inflammatory enlargement of active infection.

The exact cause of local gigantism is not known. It could be related to wound healing and various growth factors. The process of wound healing is controlled by growth factors that initiate cell growth and proliferation by binding to specific high affinity receptors on the cell surface. They have the ability to stimulate mitosis of quiescent cells. Growth factors are produced by platelets, macrophages, epithelial cells, fibroblasts, and endothelial cells. The cause of local gigantism could be because of increased sensitivity of local receptors to various growth factors or their increased production locally during the process of wound repair. Growth factors promote proliferation of endothelial cells, fibroblasts, keratinocytes and chondrocytes, and may thus lead to gigantism. The other possible mechanisms may be local arteriovenous malformations or lymphatic blockade.

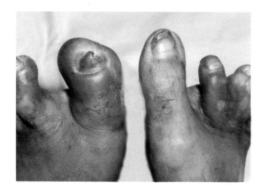

Fig. 21.1: Local gigantism of left great toe

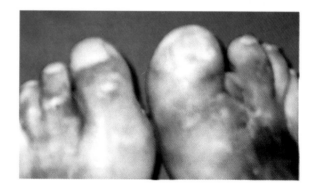

Fig. 21.2: Local gigantism of right great toe

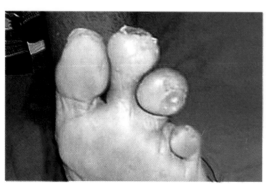

Fig. 21.3: Local gigantism 2nd and 3rd toes left foot, note amputation 4th toe

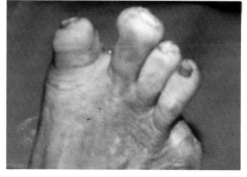

Fig. 21.4: Local gigantism of right 2nd toe, note also partial amputation 1st toe, amputation 5th toe

22 Lessons from Leprosy Foot

We owe our understanding of diabetic foot ulcers to foot ulcers of leprosy

It is interesting to note that our understanding of diabetic neuropathic foot ulcers, their management and prevention originated from experience of neuropathic foot ulcers in leprosy. It was Dr Paul Brand, who first recognized the common etiological roots that beset both diabetic and leprosy foot ulceration. His work in treating and preventing foot ulcers in leprosy, while working in India, made it possible to implement these principles in diabetic individuals.

I had the opportunity to study both, leprosy and diabetic foot cases and this chapter reveals a comparison between these two quite contrasting clinical conditions, with too palpable a socioeconomic disparity. Leprosy patients are not just poor, but are more often than not, social discards of the society, while diabetics if not most, enjoy a rather privileged social status.

Leprosy is a mutilating infective disorder caused by *Mycobacterium leprae*. Leprosy involves peripheral nerves, which are superficial subcutaneous nerves where the temperature is cooler by direct infiltration of Schwann cells by *Mycobacterium leprae*. For example posterior tibial nerve below medial malleolus, lateral popliteal nerve as it winds around the neck of fibula, ulnar nerve at the elbow, median nerve at the wrist and so on. Paralysis of these nerves leads to sensory, motor, and autonomic dysfunctions. Neuropathic foot ulcerations are akin to those in diabetics.

INVOLVEMENT OF FOOT

There are two sites where nerves affecting foot are commonly paralysed in leprosy. The first is paralysis of posterior tibial nerve, which leads to loss of sensation of the plantar aspect of foot and paralysis of the intrinsic muscles. The second site of paralysis is lateral popliteal nerve as it winds around the neck of

fibula and it leading to foot drop, loss of extensor power in the toes and also paralysis of the peroneal muscles. The affected foot is thus insensate dry and fissured (autonomic dysfunction). It is also deformed with areas of increased plantar pressures (intrinsic minus foot) and is all set for neuropathic ulcerations.

In leprosy it is interesting to see recurring and longstanding foot ulcers of duration more than 10 years, which continue to occur even after the complete cure of the disease. The chronicity of foot ulceration in leprosy is obviously because of lack of off-loading of plantar ulcers. The leprosy affected have to keep working for the sake of their daily bread with as a consequence, rest to the affected foot an unattainable luxury. I vividly recollect, as a resident in leprosy wards, the ward rounds had to be done before 8 a.m. or only after 8 p.m. as in between the patients had slipped out of their beds in search of livelihood, even if and often it was reduced to begging, capitalizing on their disfigurement and multiple leaking wounds. Another reason for chronicity of ulcerations is the bilateral feet and hand involvement. All these features clearly indicate that leprosy patients are severely physically handicapped, than patients with diabetes. The Charcot foot is extremely common in leprosy and is often bilateral. In fact, I have seen garden varieties of Charcot feet in leprosy cases (Fig. 22.1). The degree

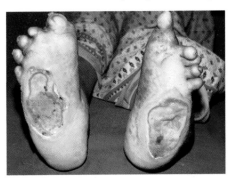

Fig. 22.1: Bilateral Charcot feet with mid foot plantar ulcers

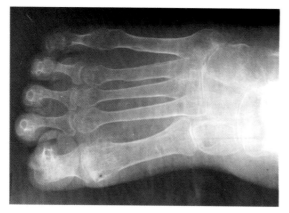

Fig. 22.2: Radiograph showing marked osteoporosis

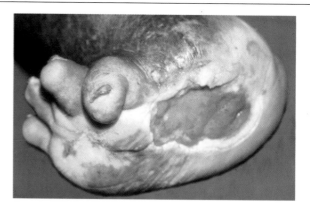

Fig. 22.3: Note clean and red floor
of the plantar ulcer

of osteopenia is extreme and the bones on radiographic examination appear almost decalcified (Fig. 22.2). Another peculiarity is a clean and red ulcer floor, (Fig. 22.3), whereas in diabetics it is often exudative, dirty and pale yellow. Maggots are natural friends of leprosy patients, who selectively remove necrotic tissue leaving the healthy tissue intact. In diabetics, the infection spreads rapidly with extensive necrosis because of underlying hyperglycemia and maggots find it difficult to keep pace.

Limb amputation in leprosy is extremely rare despite all the adverse factors. In fact one of the commonest indication for limb amputation in leprosy, is the squamous cell carcinoma which is malignant transformation of a chronic neuropathic ulcer. Chronic neuropathic ulcer is thus a precancerous condition. In diabetics the ulcers do not have such a prolonged course, extending over a decade, to get transformed into malignancy because by then either the ulcer has healed or the limb or the patient have been lost.

Table 22.1: Clinical differences between leprosy and diabetic neuropathy		
Characteristics	*Leprosy neuropathy*	*Diabetic neuropathy*
Etiology	Direct infiltration of nerves by lepra bacilli	Metabolic, microangiopathy
Type	Mononeuropathy multiplex	Diffuse polyneuropathy
Nerves affected	Superficial nerves where temperature is cooler and not length related	Length related (long nerves) are involved
Bilateral feet lesions	Very common	Common
Bilateral hand lesions	Very common	Rare
Charcot foot	Very common > 35%	Less common <10%
Peripheral nerves	Thick and tender	Slightly thick non-tender
Malignancy in chronic ulcer	Does occur	Never
Limb amputation	Rare	Common

Despite all adverse factors, such as socioeconomic status, increased biomechanical stress, continued weight bearing, bilateral feet involvement, severe physical disabilities and lack of access to expert healthcare, limb amputations are significantly less common in leprosy patients. The clinical course of leprosy foot lesion is a slow progressive destruction, autoamputations associated with restructuring and remodelling of the feet (Figs 22.4 A to 22.5B). The feet are still walkable despite their marked shortening. On the other hand, despite shorter duration of foot lesions, access to expert healthcare and a relatively better socioeconomic status, the clinical course of infected foot lesion in diabetics is rapid deterioration, requiring limb amputations more frequently. Chronic hyperglycemia and vascular insufficiency stand out as the two most important detrimental factors in diabetes.

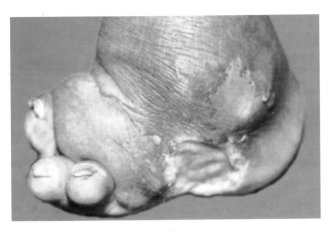

Fig. 22.4A: Walkable foot with remodelling and autoamputation almost like a Lisfranc amputation but with toes

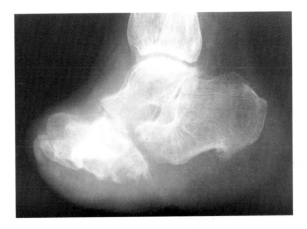

Fig. 22.4B: Radiograph showing absorption of metatarsals and phalanges, note Charcot foot at the ankle joint

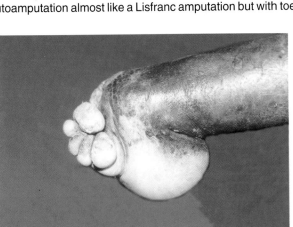

Fig. 22.5A: Walkable foot with remodelling and auto-amputation almost like a Chopart amputation but with toes

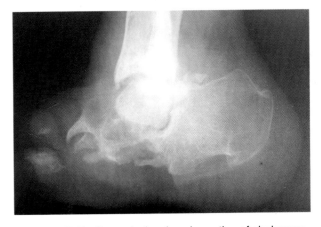

Fig. 22.5B: Radiograph showing absorption of phalanges, metatarsals and tarsal bones. Note Charcot foot at the ankle joint

23 Plantar Ulcers, Management Principles

*Antibiotics and dressings do not heal plantar ulcers,
It is the off-loading that heals them!*

Plantar ulcers are probably the greatest concern while treating a diabetic patient. This ulceration is most commonly a continuum of a callus that went unrecognized and untreated. The importance of identification of the plantar ulcer and ensuring its healing is of paramount importance. It is the forerunner of destructive lesions of the foot eventually requiring a limb amputation. It is important to realize that, 85% of leg amputations are preceded by foot ulceration. The plantar ulcerations can occur at any site, governed mainly by an area of increased pressure. The common sites are ball of the great toe, plantar aspects of the heads of the metatarsals, tips of the toes, the lateral border of the foot and heel. The mid foot is usually spared as it is mostly non-weight bearing. However, midfoot ulceration is a characteristic feature of the Charcot foot.

EVALUATION OF THE PLANTAR ULCER

A proper evaluation of a plantar ulcer is a prerequisite for planning management strategies. A plantar ulcer should be evaluated from various angles described below.

Site of the Ulcer

There is a close association of the location of an ulcer and its etiology, e.g. a mid foot ulceration with the Charcot foot, a toe ulceration with the hammer toe deformity.

Size of the Ulcer

It is important to measure the dimensions of the ulcer to determine the duration of wound healing and monitor its progress. The correct size of an ulcer can be determined only after debridement of its margins (Fig. 23.1).

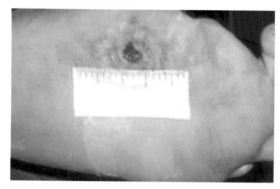

Fig. 23.1: Size of the ulcer determined after debridement

Depth of the Ulcer

The depth of an ulcer decides the prognosis and severity of the lesion. The prognosis of an ulcer is directly proportional to its depth. This can be measured by inserting a sterile metallic probe into the ulcer (Fig. 23.2). Probing also helps in the diagnosis of osteomyelitis of the underlying bone. If the metallic probe penetrates to bone, it confirms the diagnosis of an osteomyelitis.

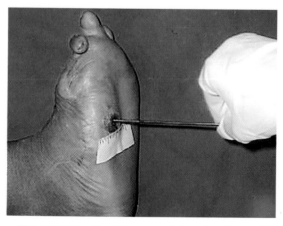

Fig. 23.2: Depth of the ulcer determined by probing

Floor of the Ulcer

One should know whether the ulcer floor is granular or necrotic, exudative (discharging) or dry and foul smelling or otherwise (Figs 23.3 and 23.4).

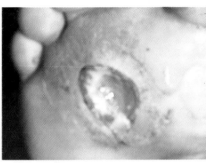

Fig. 23.3: Floor of the ulcer exudative (discharging)

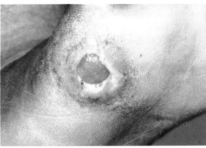

Fig. 23.4: Granulating floor of the ulcer

Margins of the Ulcer

Margins of the ulcer are often hyperkeratotic. They can also be undermined, adherent, macerated or necrotic (Figs 23.5 and 23.6).

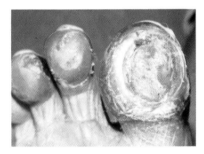

Fig. 23.5: Hyperkeratotic margins of the ulcer

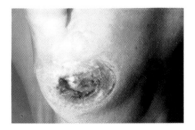

Fig. 23.6: Necrotic margins of the ulcer

Presence of Infection

It is essential to ascertain whether the ulcer is infected. Appropriate microbial cultures and radiographs are necessary for the diagnosis of osteomyelitis and planning of the appropriate antibiotic therapy.

Presence of Ischemia

The plantar ulcers are usually not associated with ischemia. However, it is mandatory to palpate the peripheral pulses and measure ABI.

Contralateral Foot

After an examination of the ulcerated foot, it is essential to examine the other foot. It is this foot, which will have to bear most of the body weight in order to rest the ulcerated one.

MANAGEMENT PRINCIPLES

It is now well recognized that the primary factor in the cause of diabetic plantar ulcer is the presence of an insensate foot due to neuropathy. This insensitivity allows excessive and prolonged stress and pressures to occur in the diabetic foot, which ultimately results in tissue breakdown. If the tissue breakdown (ulcer) goes unnoticed or untreated, an infection is imminent and major amputation is likely. If the ulceration is the result of an increased plantar pressure, the treatment should focus on reducing this pressure at the ulcer site. This relief of pressure can be achieved mainly by mechanical control (off-loading), and by resting the affected foot.

OFF-LOADING

Ideally the plantar ulcers must be managed with rest and avoidance of pressure. Total non-weight bearing (bed-rest) is neither practical nor acceptable to most of the patients. Various other methods of off-loading are discussed below in brief.

- *Wheel chair :* A light weight folding wheel chair can be of great help in achieving maximal off-loading (Fig. 23.7). It is especially useful if the ulcers are bilateral or infected.
- *Crutches:* This is an inexpensive and one of the most practical methods of off-loading (Fig. 23.8). The

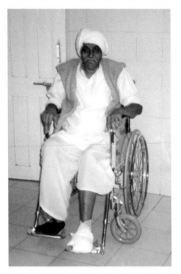

Fig. 23.7: Use of wheel chair for off-loading

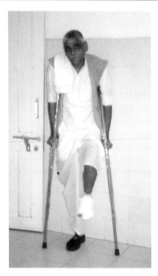

Fig. 23.8: Use of crutches for off-loading

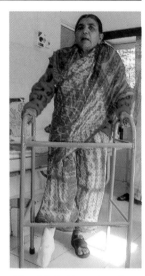

Fig. 23.9: Use of walker for off-loading

greatest advantage is ability to attend work. However, elderly patients and patients with amyotrophy find it difficult to walk with hand held crutches. It is important to train the patient for their proper use to avoid falls and accidents, especially on the stairs. The unaffected foot should be regularly inspected as the risk of ulceration is increased because of extra weight bearing. The use of crutches is particularly useful for patients with an infected ulcer, which needs regular dressing.

- *Walker:* A light weight metallic folding walker provides stability and is a good alternative for patients who cannot cope with the crutches (Fig. 23.9).

- *Orthopedic scooter:* This device consists of a metal frame attached to a trolley with four small wheels and an adjustable-height padded channel on which the patient can rest their lower leg and foot while propelling themselves with the contralateral foot.

- *Total contact cast (TCC):* It is the "Gold standard" among various methods used to aid the healing of plantar foot ulcers. The principle of TCC is to equalize loading of the plantar surface by a uniform "total contact" of the plantar surface with the cast material thereby increasing the weight-bearing area and minimizing the pressure at the ulcer site. Different steps in encasing the affected foot in a TCC are shown (Figs 23.10 to 23.12). It is important to "pad" the ulcer area with soft foam before putting the cast on, in order to create void under

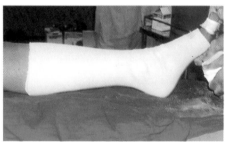

Fig. 23.10: Stockinette is rolled over the foot and leg

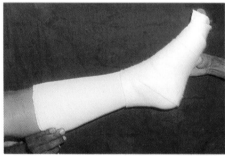

Fig. 23.11: A layer of cotton padding is applied

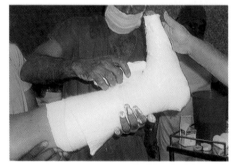

Fig. 23.12: A layer of plaster is continuously molded around the bony prominences until it has set

the ulcer. Plantar pressure studies have shown a reduction in the pressure at the ulcer site with TCC by over 80%. Most of the ulcers heal in approximately 6 weeks. See case study 23.B (Fig. 23.22A to C).

Indication

Non-infected plantar ulcer.

Contraindications

Absolute:
• Infected plantar ulcer
• Non-compliant patient
Relative:
• Ulcer depth greater than its width
• Swelling of the foot
• ABI 0.5 or less

The patients should be instructed for proper care of the cast and to report immediately if there is pain, discomfort, swelling or fever. There are usually no major problems with TCC if properly applied. However some patients find it too heavy and uncomfortable. The other disadvantages are an inability to drive a vehicle, disuse atrophy of the muscles, osteoporosis, and joint stiffness.

• *Air cast:* This is a bi-valve cast, the two halves being joined together with a Velcro strapping. The air cast is lined with four air cells, which can be inflated with a hand pump through four valves to ensure a close fit. The cast is removable so that the patients can check their ulcers and remove the cast when in bed (Fig. 23.13).

• *Temporary shoes:* Whenever it is not possible to provide a cast, a readymade temporary shoe with

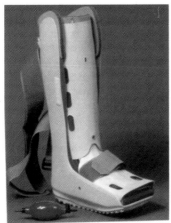

Fig. 23.13: Air cast *(courtesy M. E Edmonds & AVM Foster, King's College Hospital, London, UK)*

cushioned insole can be provided (Figs 23.14 and 23.15). The shoe is of a universal size and is large enough to accommodate the dressing. The shoe shape is such that it can be worn in either in the left or the right foot. Once the ulcer has healed, the same shoe can be worn by another patient. The patient must be made to realize that the activity level should be minimum.

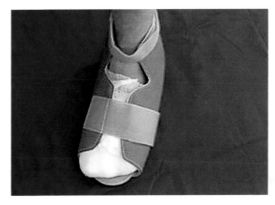

Fig. 23.14: Darco shoe

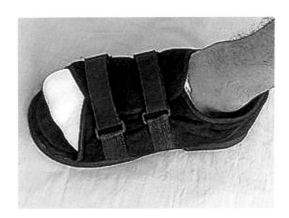

Fig. 23.15: Temporary shoe

• *Felt and foam dressings:* This approach consists of adhering bilayer of felt and foam to the patient's foot, foam being in contact with the skin. An area of pressure relief is created by removing the foam and felt layer from the vulnerable ulcer area, thus transferring the load to the other areas. An extra depth shoe is worn to accommodate the bulk of the dressing.

• *Weight relief shoes (half shoes):* These shoes offer support only under the rear and mid foot leaving the forefoot "suspended" and hence are useful to help healing of the forefoot ulcers. They effectively off-load the area being treated, instead of simply redistributing the pressures (Figs 23.16 and 23.17). They must be individually fitted and modified as necessary, to ensure an effective and safe fit.

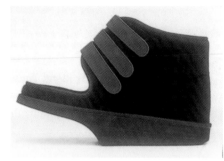

Fig. 23.16: Half shoe (Reproduced with kind permission of the "international working group on the diabetic foot")

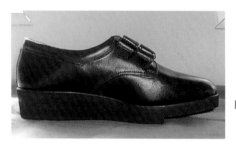

Fig. 23.17: Forefoot relief shoe

- *Plantar metatarsal pads:* They are modified insoles, which are stuck on the plain insole and inserted inside the extra depth footwear (Fig. 23.18). They help in redistributing weight bearing away from the vulnerable ulcer site (under metatarsal head). They are wide enough to cover the whole forefoot, are two-third of the length of the metatarsal and end just before the toes. These pads are 8 mm in thickness. The area of the ulcer is cut out so as to suspend the ulcer. The edges of the cut out area (wing) are bevelled. These pads are useful for superficial plantar ulcers on toes and underneath the metatarsal heads.

- *Molded insoles:* They are designed to redistribute the pressure and to provide cushioning. A plaster of Paris cast of the foot is taken to represent its overall contours including the sole. The cast is filled with a foam to make a last, over which the insoles are molded. They can be made of microcellular rubber, ethyl-vinyl-acetate (EVA) or polyethylene foam. The composite insoles can be made using different foams, the upper layer consists of a low density closed cell polyethylene foam such as plastazote (Fig. 23.19). These closed cell materials do not absorb fluids and can be easily cleaned and therefore be used in contact with the wound surface. Open cell materials, such as poron is used as a lower layer to provide shock absorption and shear reduction.

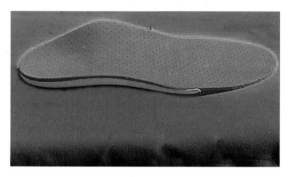

Fig. 23.19: Composite insole

- *Winged outsole:* We have found outsole modification equally useful as insole modifications. The molded insoles are difficult to make, cannot be inspected inside the shoes and there is always a risk of the ulcer margins crossing the window or void; while outsole modifications are easy to make, can be inspected and last longer (Fig. 23.20). An inch (2.5 cm) thick rigid rubber sole is stuck to the existing outer sole of the footwear. A sole of similar

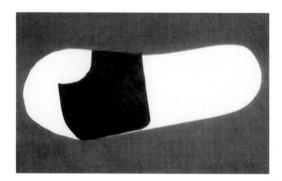

Fig. 23.18: Plantar metatarsal pad (PMP)

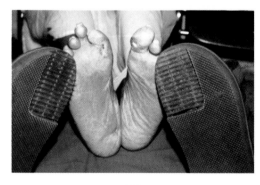

Fig. 23.20: Winged outsole

thickness is stuck to the other footwear so as to equalize the length. The vulnerable area can be suspended by cutting the wing of the outsole.

Total contact casting (TCC) is the most effective and scientifically studied method of off-loading. The other methods are either anecdotal or have been tried only on a small number of patients. During the process of off-loading using any of the methods described above, care should be taken that the ulcer cavity should not be packed as this would inhibit healing of the ulcer. The techniques of off-loading can only succeed if the patient is committed to refraining from ever putting the affected foot on the ground unprotected. If an ulcer does not show adequate progress to healing, a specialist referral is recommended.

Off-loading should be continued until the ulcer has healed completely, plus two more weeks to permit maturation of the wound. Off-loading and a graduated return to the weight bearing in a proper footwear, may reduce the chances of the development of an acute neuro-arthropathic process or recurrence of the ulcer. Ongoing evaluation of the contralateral extremity is also essential. The chances of a fresh ulceration on contralateral limb are increased because of extra weight bearing.

Off-Loading Bilateral Plantar Ulcers

This is the most difficult situation. Most of the methods described above cannot be used in presence of bilateral ulcers. If the ulcers are deep, they must be rested, either in the bed or by use of a wheel chair. Once the depth and size of the ulcers are reduced, weight relief shoes and molded insoles can be provided. The most important aspect in bilateral plantar ulcerations is to reduce the activity level to a minimum possible.

PREVENTION OF RECURRENCE

A recurrent foot wound is defined as any tissue breakdown at the same site as the original ulcer that occurs in >30 days from the time of original healing. Any new tissue breakdown within 30 days of healing at the same site is considered as part of the original episode. A wound at a different site is considered to be a new episode whenever the wound occurs.

The prevention of recurrence of a plantar ulcer is a much more difficult task than its healing. A recurrence of a chronic plantar ulcer is the rule unless preventive

steps such as a life-long surveillance and continued pressure relief measures are undertaken. This is caused by a lack of strict non-weight bearing in spite of the various modalities of off-loading. It is virtually impossible for the patient to avoid walking altogether bearing weight on the affected limb. The patients need to be educated regarding non-weight bearing in every situation they may encounter in day-to-day living. Even few steps a day on the affected foot can delay healing.

ROLE OF SURGERY

In chronic recurrent indolent plantar ulcers, surgery is recommended especially for the forefoot ulcers. It involves removal of one or all the metatarsal heads through the dorsum of the foot (Figs 23.28A to G). See case study 23.H.

NEWER THERAPIES

Regranex gel (platelet derived growth factor), bio-engineered human dermis (Dermagraft), Apligraf are some of the recent therapies, which have been found to be effective in promoting healing of non-infected plantar ulcers. They are discussed in detail in a separate chapter No. 48.

Case Study (23.A)

This 54 years old male, a bank employee, with type 2 DM of 12 years, presented with bilateral plantar ulcers. He had an ulcer on the 1st MTH of left foot and another infected ulcer on the 3rd MTH of right foot, which was 2.5 cm in diameter and depth. He also had an infected ulcer on the dorsomedial aspect of the right great toe with osteomyelitis of the terminal phalanx (Fig. 23.21 A). He had already undergone 2nd toe disarticulation of the left foot resulting in hallux valgus

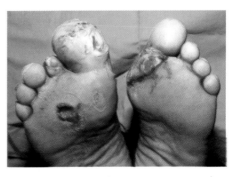

Fig. 23.21A: Bilateral feet ulcers on 1st MTH (left), ulcers on 3rd MTH and great toe (right)

and a partial 2nd toe amputation of the right foot. In view of bilateral ulcerations, he was advised bed rest for two weeks and intravenous antibiotics for the first week followed by oral antibiotics for 6 weeks. The surgical debridement of all the 3 ulcers was carried out simultaneously, on admission. The terminal phalanx of the right great toe was removed. His left foot ulcer healed faster as it was superficial. He was then given crutches to offload the right foot and temporary forefoot pressure relief shoe for left foot. At the end of 2 months, his feet were ulcer free (Fig. 23.21B). He was advised forefoot pressure relief footwear and to reduce his activities to bare minimum.

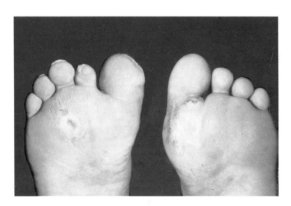

Fig. 23.21B: Bilateral ulcers healed in 2 months

Case Study (23.B)

This 45 years old male, an agriculturist, with type 2 DM of 20 years had history of recurrent ulceration on the left foot, ball of the great toe, for last six years. He had undergone skin grafting, 3 years ago, which never worked. The present ulcer, at the same site, was non-healing since last 9 months (Fig. 23.22A). There was no evidence of osteomyelitis or infection. He was given TCC. The ulcer healed in 6 weeks (Figs 23.22B and C). He has now been advised to reduce his activity level and forefoot pressure relief shoes for outdoors and sandals for indoors to prevent the recurrence.

In the last 6 years he was hospitalized several times, elsewhere, for the treatment of recurrent plantar ulcer. This time he was treated ambulatory, with excellent results. For the last 6 months it has not recurred.

Case Study (23.C)

This 67 years old male, with type 2 DM of 24 years presented with non-healing ulcer on the left foot 1st

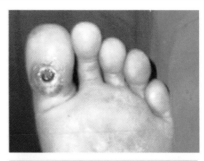

Fig. 23.22A: Ulcer on ball of the great toe (left)

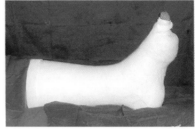

Fig. 23.22B: TCC applied for six weeks after removing the callus

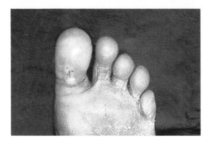

Fig. 23.22C: Ulcer has almost healed

MTH since 2 years. The ulcer was small, 0.5 cm in diameter and superficial; it was not infected. The ulcer was cleaned and the patient was given extra depth shoes with soft insoles and left plantar metatarsal pad (Figs 23.23A to C). The ulcer healed in 6 weeks and the patient has remained ulcer free for 4 years, when

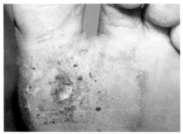

Fig. 23.23A: Superficial ulcer on 1st MTH left foot

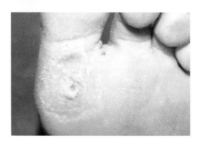

Fig. 23.23B: Healing ulcer

he was last seen. However his 3D scan continued to show increased plantar pressure on 1st MTH left foot (Fig. 23.23D). Extra depth shoe, PMP and reduced activity have helped in preventing the recurrence.

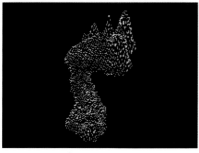

Fig. 23.23C: Ulcer healed with PMP and extradepth shoes

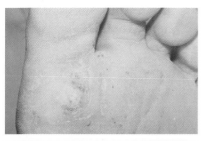

Fig. 23.23D: 3D scan showing increased plantar pressure on 1st MTH, & hallux left foot

Case Study (23.D)

This 53 years old lady, an office clerk, with type 2 DM of 16 years, presented with non-healing ulcer on plantar aspect of the left great toe, since 2 years (Fig. 23.24A). The ulcer was 2 cm in diameter and 1 cm deep. There was no osteomyelitis. Under antibiotics' cover, the ulcer was debrided. She was advised bed rest for one week and was gradually allowed ambulation using crutches. The antibiotics were continued for 2 weeks. Since she had to resume her duties, she was given left plantar metatarsal pad and extra depth shoes, as crutches were not acceptable in the office. The ulcer healed completely in 2 months (Figs 23.24B and C).

Case Study (23.E)

This 62 years old male with type 2 DM of 18 years, with renal insufficiency presented with an active ulcer on the right foot near the base of great toe and a history of recurrent ulcer on the left great toe plantar aspect. After cleaning of the ulcers, the patient was advised outsole modification. The right foot ulcer healed in 6 weeks and the ulcer on left great toe never recurred during followup period of 2 years (Figs 23.25A to D).

Case Study (23.F)

This 65 years old lady presented with an ulcer over plantar aspect of the left great toe. The ulcer was

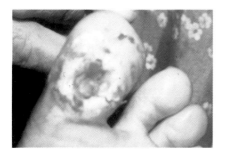

Fig. 23.24A: Non-healing ulcer left great toe

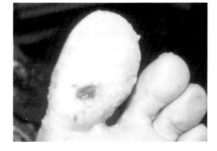

Fig. 23.24B: Ulcer healing with use of crutches

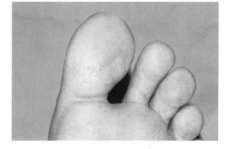

Fig. 23.24C: Ulcer healed with PMP and extradepth shoe

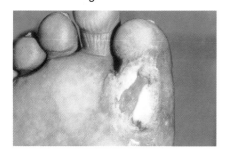

Fig. 23.25A: Ulcer over right great toe

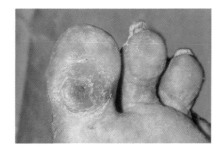

Fig. 23.25B: Callosity left great toe, site of recurrent ulceration

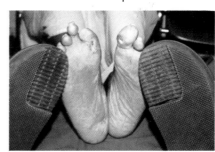

Fig. 23.25C: Use of winged outsoles

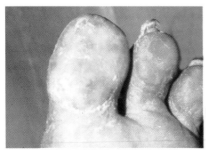

Fig. 23.25D: Left great toe ulcer never recurred

occupying the ball of the great toe, was superficial with red granulating floor (Fig. 23.26A) and did not have any evidence of infection. History revealed that she had injured her great toe and had developed swelling with a blister. Surgical debridement and deroofing of the blister was carried out elsewhere, one and half months ago. Despite good surgery, the wound was not healing. The treating surgeon was giving her cefuroxime for the last 6 weeks and the wound dressing was being carried out every day at his clinic. The lady had to walk about half a mile (one kilometer) for the daily dressing and this was the cause for non-healing of the ulcer. We advised her to stop antibiotics, and get the dressings done at home. In 4 weeks, the wound healed completely (Fig. 23.26B). Non-weight bearing is extremely important, when the ulcer is active.

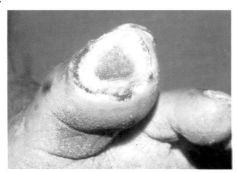

Fig. 23.26A: Non-healing ulcer left great toe

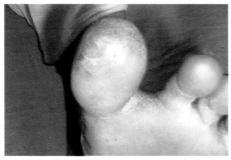

Fig. 23.26B: Ulcer healed in 4 weeks with off-loading

Case Study (23.G)

This 64 years old lady, wife of a doctor, with type 2 DM of 32 years, had insensate feet with gross deformities of all the toes. She was a regular visitor at our foot clinic for frequent ulcerations and callus removals (Figs 23.27A and B). For two long years, she did not turn up and I wondered what had happened to her. One fine day she came to our clinic, I was curious to see her feet! And to my great surprise, although deformed, her feet were ulcer free. I hesitantly enquired as to where she was being treated so well. She had not received treatment from elsewhere, she said. Further enquiry revealed that she was earlier staying in a ground floor apartment wherefrom she used to go outdoors frequently. For the last 2 years, they had shifted to a 4th floor apartment which had no elevator. Because of severe osteoarthritis of her knees, she was going out of her home only on her birthday. The cause of non-recurrence of the ulcers was a drastic reduction in the activity level (Fig. 23.27 C). However, 3D scan revealed areas of increased plantar pressure (Fig. 23.27 D). For

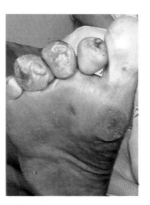

Fig. 23.27A: Callus on 1st MTH and tips of toes right foot

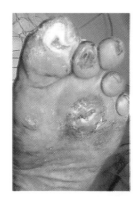

Fig. 23.27B: Ulcer on great toe 3rd MTH, toe deformities left foot

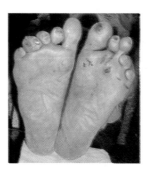

Fig. 23.27C: Two years later, active ulcers and callus growth minimal

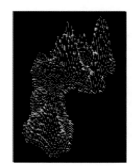

Fig. 23.27D: 3D scan shows multiple areas of increased plantar pressure

the plantar ulcers to occur, it is important to have sensory neuropathy with LOPS, increased plantar pressure and continued weight bearing (increased activity level). In this case, feet did not ulcerate because of reduced activity level, although first two factors were still operating.

Case Study (23.H)

This 74 years old male with type 2 DM of 25 years duration presented with a non-healing plantar ulcers on right foot, one near the base of 5th toe since 3 years, with intermittent recurrence and another close to the base of 2nd toe, since 1 year. Both the ulcers discharged pus off and on. He was hospitatized several times and had received antibiotics for a prolonged period, contact plaster cast and had also undergone debridements of the ulcers. His general and systemic examinations were normal with BP 130/80 mmHg. Local examination revealed neuropathic feet with normal ABI. He had an ulcer over the 2nd MTH measuring 4 cm in length, 2.5 cm in width and 3 cm in depth. However, probing did not reveal any evidence of osteomyelitis. The ulcer over the 5th MTH was 3 cm in length, 2 cm wide and 3 cm deep. Probing revealed evidence of osteomyelitis. There was purulent discharge from both the ulcers (Figs 23.28A and B).

He was hospitalized and started on to broad spectrum I/V antibiotics, insulin therapy and investigated. His Hb 10.5 gms%, TLC 10,000/cu.mm,

ESR 121 mm/1st hr, S. Creatinine 1.1 mg/dL plasma glucose 168 mg% and HbA$_1$c 6.1% He had early background retinopathy left eye and blindness of the right eye secondary to failed cataract surgery. His resting ECG showed T wave inversion in V5 and V6. 2D Echocardiography was normal, X-ray of the right foot showed evidence of osteomyelitis of the 5th metatarsal (Fig. 23.28C).

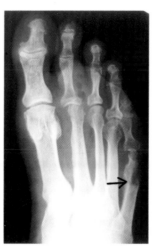

Fig. 23.28C: Radiograph showing osteomyelitis of 5th metatarsal (right)

In view of a prolonged history of recurrent ulceration on 2nd MTH and osteomyelitis of the 5th metatarsal, he was subjected to condylectomy of 2nd MT head through dorsal approach and a partial excision of the 5th metatarsal along with the 5th MT head (Figs 23.28 D and E) through lateral border of the foot (non-weight bearing area). Both the ulcers

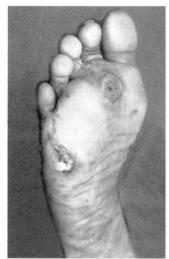

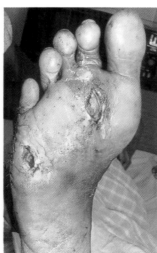

Fig. 23.28A: Plantar ulcers with thick callus, maceration and discharge

Fig. 23.28B: After callus removal the measurements were taken

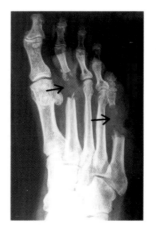

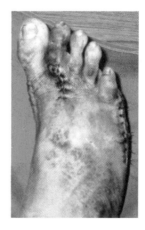

Fig. 23.28D: Radiograph showing partial resection of 5th metatarsal and 2nd and 5th MT heads (condylectomy)

Fig. 23.28E: Condylectomy and resection of 5th metatarsal carried out through non-weight bearing areas

were debrided and bacterial culture sent from the deeper tissues. However, cultures did not reveal growth of any organisms. The patient was advised ambulation using a walker as he had a difficulty balancing on the crutches. IV antibiotics were continued for 2 weeks and was later on switched on to cefuroxime 250 mg twice daily. In four weeks, the size of the ulcers had reduced significantly, with no purulent discharge (Figs 23.28F and 23.28G).

In patients with chronic non healing plantar ulcers with recurrent infection, surgical removal of one or more metatarsal heads, should be considered as an option, if all other measures of off-loading have failed. The metatarsal heads are removed by a dorsal approach to avoid injury to the plantar skin (weight bearing area).

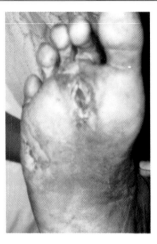

Fig. 23.28F: After 2 weeks, note reduction in size of the ulcers

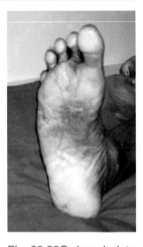

Fig. 23.28G: 4 weeks later, the ulcers have almost healed

SectionThree

Nail and Skin Lesions

- Nail Lesions

- Diabetic Dermopathy

- Necrobiosis Lipoidica Diabeticorum

24 Nail Lesions

Nail is an asset, a protective toe cap
In high-risk foot, it is often a liability

Nails are natural appendages of skin and protect toes from extrinsic trauma. They are normally cut and trimmed regularly by every individual. However diabetics with advanced age, diminished vision, and central obesity find it difficult to see and reach toe nails. Hence while cutting even the normal nails, they tend to cut the soft tissue causing injury and ulceration.

In neuropathic patients with or without ischemia, nails are often thickened, dystrophic, deformed, and are afflicted with fungal infection. Nail of the great toe is commonly affected, but any toe nail may be involved. Such nails are difficult to cut by usual nail cutter and should be regularly cut and trimmed by a podiatrist. The common nail lesions are discussed below.

Onychomycosis

Fungal infections are normally found in the hyperhydrotic foot or after nail trauma. Diabetic neuropathy leads to nail trauma with subsequent subungual hemorrhage increasing the risk of fungal infection. The nails are discoloured and the nail plate is usually whitish or yellowish; the normal glistening appearance is replaced by a dull and splintered one (Fig. 24.1). The fungus actually invades the nailbed, infecting the nail as it grows distally. The nail is hypertrophied, multilayered and disorganized as it grows out and separates from the nailbed distally. Eradication of the fungal infection in such dystrophic nails is extremely difficult. Regular trimming of the nails and reducing the bulk should be carried out by a podiatrist. Local and systemic antifungal agents should also be given.

Onychocryptosis (Ingrowing Toe Nail)

They have an excessive lateral curvature and trap epithelial cells in the sulcus and pinch the nailbed, making it painful. Inadequate nail cutting or digging down the side of the sulcus, to remove debris, often leaves behind a splinter of the nail which grows forward and penetrates the nail sulcus (Figs 24.2 and 24.3). The sulcus should be gently cleared with a file; removal of the edge of the nail is also helpful. Partial nail removal or total matrixectomy are often required in patients with a severe problem.

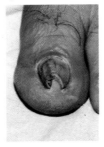

Fig. 24.2: Ingrowing toe nail (onychocryptosis)

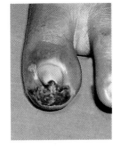

Fig. 24.3: Ingrowing toe nail has led to ulceration and hemorrhage

Onychogryphosis (Thickened Nails)

Thickened nails are extremely common in long standing diabetics with neuropathy with or without

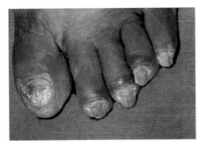

Fig. 24.1: Onychomycosis

ischemia. Excess of keratin and debris accumulate under the nail and in the nail folds (Figs 24.4 and 24.5). Bulk of the nail should be regularly reduced, else the shoe will press on the thickened nail plate and cause a subungual ulcer (Fig. 24.6). Excess debris can become a nidus for bacterial infection.

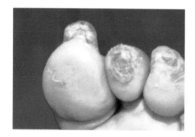

Fig. 24.4: Thickened nail left great toe (onychogryphosis)

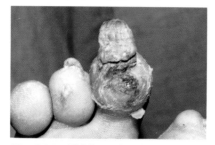

Fig. 24.5: Thickened nail with ulcer on tip of the 2nd toe

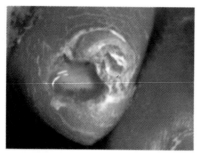

Fig. 24.6: Subungual ulcer *(Courtesy ME Edmonds and AVM Foster, King's College Hospital, London, UK)*

Onychauxis (Deformed Nails)

The nails are thickened and deformed. The cause is an insult to the nailbed, the result being irregular nail growth (Figs 24.7 to 24.9). Deformed nails should be regularly cut using a nail clipper, by a podiatrist, as they otherwise grow at an angle and penetrate the adjacent toes, producing ulceration. These crooked nails get caught in socks or bed clothes and cause trauma to the nailbed.

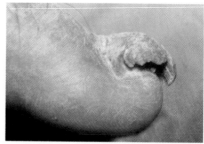

Fig. 24.7: Beak-like nail

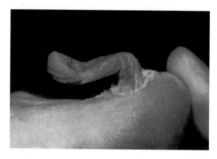

Fig. 24.8: Ram's horn, deformed nail (onychauxis) *(Courtesy ME Edmonds and AVM Foster, King's College Hospital, London, UK)*

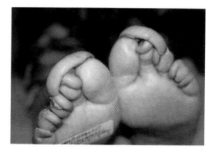

Fig. 24.9: Grossly deformed nails both feet (with permission, international working group on the diabetic foot)

Paronychia

It is the bacterial infection of the nailbed, associated with an inflammatory swelling on the sides of the nail. A pressure on the nailbed, drains purulent material (Figs 24.10 and 24.11). It has been attributed to several factors including trauma, nail dystrophy, ill-fitting shoes, and improper nail cutting. Antibiotics followed by adequate conservative debridement of the offending border should be implemented with a close continued follow-up of the patient. However, if the infection continues, the offending border may be removed by partial matrixectomy, and if both the borders are involved, by total matrixectomy. Careful evaluation of the vascular status is essential before such a surgery.

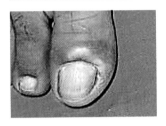

Fig. 24.10: Paronychia, note the small abscess

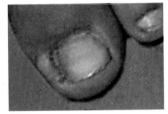

Fig. 24.11: Paronychia, note the small abscess

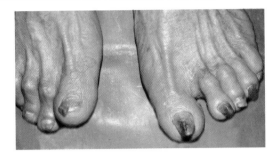

Fig. 24.13A: Dystrophic nails

Subungual Hematoma

This is usually seen secondary to trauma. Hemorrhage can be seen underneath the nail (Fig. 24.12). If left untreated, this hematoma can be a nidus for bacterial infection and subungual ulceration. Usually, the nail is already avulsed due to trauma. The nail needs to be removed under antibiotic coverage.

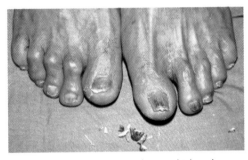

Fig. 24.13B: After cutting and trimming

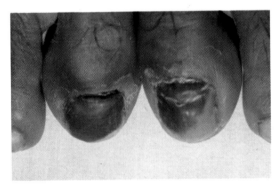

Fig. 24.12: Hemorrhage underneath the nails of both great toes

Regular Care of Nails

Patients with thickened and deformed nails, so also patients with diminished vision, old age, need regular nail care by a podiatrist using nail clipper and nail files. These nails should be cut across using a nail clipper, should be trimmed and filed (Figs 24.13A to 24.15). Excess bulk of the nail should be periodically reduced.

Patients with normal nails, good vision and those who have been adequately taught about nail cutting should be instructed to :
- Cut nails after bath, when they are soft.
- Do not try to cut the entire nail in one piece
- Do not cut nails too short.
- Never cut the corner of the nail or dig down its sides.

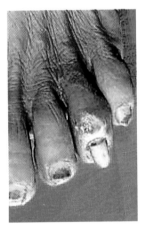

Fig. 24.14A: Partially avulsed nail, with ulcer on dorsum of left 4th toe due to ill-fitting shoe

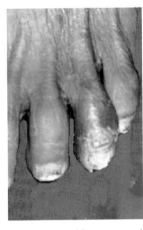

Fig. 24.14B: After removal of the nail

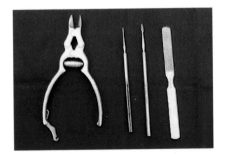

Fig. 24.15: Nail clipper and nail files

25 Diabetic Dermopathy

A cutaneous marker of diabetes

Diabetic dermopathy is characterized by circumscribed brown circular patches of 10 to 12 mm in diameter, seen on the tibial shin in diabetic subjects. They are also referred to as **Melin's shin spots**.

They are caused by minor skin trauma and may represent an altered reaction to trauma. The etiology of such lesions is unknown, though they have been closely associated with posttraumatic atrophy and postinflammatory hyperpigmentation in poorly vascularized skin. These lesions never ulcerate. The prevalence of these lesions increases with the age and duration of diabetes and correlate with the micro-angiopathies. They are seen in both type 1 and types 2 diabetics and they are twice as common in men as in women.

The lesions are at first small, dull red, scaly papules and small plaques. They eventuate to the characteristic, multiple, bilateral circumscribed, round or oval, shallow, pigmented (brown) scars on peritibial areas (Figs 25.1 and 25.2). Diabetic dermopathy being asymptomatic, requires no treatment except for protection from trauma. In Indian context, common trauma in backfiring of a two wheeler starter kick.

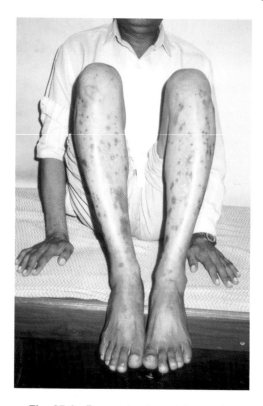

Fig. 25.1: Brown circular patches on both tibial shins in a 54 years old male

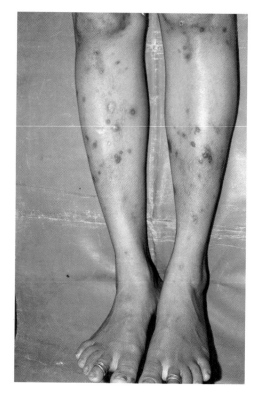

Fig. 25.2: Melin's shin spots of diabetic dermopathy on tibial shin in a 56 years old female

26 Necrobiosis Lipoidica Diabeticorum

Ulcerated lesions do not heal so easily

Necrobiosis lipoidica diabeticorum (NLD) is a cutaneous marker of diabetes and a relatively rare condition seen in less than 1% of patients. NLD often precedes diabetes, sometimes by several years. It is characteristically more common in women.

Most common site is tibial shin, rarely they are seen on the other parts of the body. They can be bilateral. The characteristic lesion of necrobiosis lipoidica diabeticorum is a slow enlarging irregularly contoured plaque. The border is often elevated and has a reddish periphery; the central portion at first erythematous, later becomes yellow or sclerotic and has a shiny appearance. The plaque often atrophies and is brown in color (Fig. 26.1). Lesions vary in size from a few millimeters to several centimeters. One-third of the lesions ulcerate, sometimes spontaneously and sometimes as a result of trauma. Ulcerated lesions take months to heal and often recur (Figs 26.2 and 26.3).

Although, the exact cause is not known, proposed causative factors are microangiopathy, obliterative endarteritis, immune mediated vasculitis, and non-enzymatic glycosylation. Histopathological features of NLD are characteristic. These are degeneration of collagen throughout the dermis, histocytes around the degenerated collagen, and obliterative granulomatous vasculitis.

Management

In non-ulcerated lesions no specific treatment is required except for avoidance of trauma. In ulcerative lesions, topical or intraregional steroids are to some extent effective. Aspirin, dipyridamole, pentoxifylline have been also tried with marginal success. When conservative treatment fails, radical excision followed by skin grafting is the only therapeutic option.

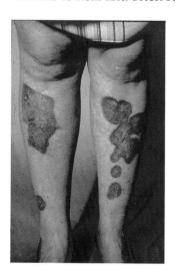

Fig. 26.1: Showing brown plaques of NLD

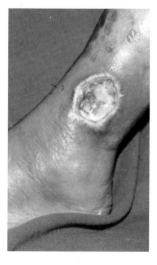

Fig. 26.2: Ulcerated lesion of NLD above lateral malleolus

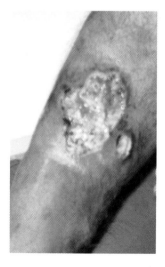

Fig. 26.3: Ulcerated lesion of NLD over tibial shin

Section Four

Infected Neuropathic Foot

- Etiopathogenesis and Diagnosis of Foot Infection

- Non-Limb Threatening Infection

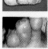

- Management of Non-Limb Threatening Infection

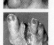

- Limb Threatening Infection

- Management of Limb Threatening Infection

- Necrotizing Fascitis

- Life Threatening Infection

27 Etiopathogenesis and Diagnosis of Foot Infection

It is the nose and not the eyes
which brings foot infection to notice

Infection of soft tissues and parenchymal organs are more common and are often more severe in diabetic patients. Foot infections are probably the most common and important of these infections. Diabetic foot infections are a serious medical problem, requiring prompt attention, appropriate diagnostic evaluation and proper therapeutic strategies. These infections are associated with longterm morbidity, bone involvement and the need for surgical debridement and amputations. In fact, diabetic foot infection is one of the commonest indications for hospitalization and prolonged hospital stays. In the beginning diabetic foot infection may appear trivial, but it has a potential to progress to limb or even life threatening situations, if not managed properly. Infection in diabetic foot works as a catalyst and accelerates the journey towards a leg amputation. Presence of ischemia has an adverse effect on the clinical course and the outcome of an infection. The combination of ischemia and infection carry the worst prognosis.

EARLY LESIONS

As long as the skin of the foot is intact, infection usually does not occur. The initial event is a break in the skin followed by penetration of microorganisms. The ulceration can be because of extrinsic factors such as mechanical trauma like stepping on sharp objects or gouging the skin while trimming nails, thermal trauma, walking barefoot, ill-fitting shoes or intrinsic factors which elevate plantar pressure and eventually lead to plantar ulceration such as limited joint mobility, callus, deformities, etc.

DORSAL FOOT INFECTION

It is relatively less common as compared to plantar foot infection. Dorsal foot infections occur mainly because of extrinsic factors and rarely progress to limb threatening situations. Unlike plantar infection, dorsal foot infection even though painless is rapidly recognized because it is visible and thus receives prompt and early medical attention (Fig. 27.1). Dorsal skin is not fixed to the underlying tissue, and can glide 2 to 3 cm. In presence of infection, the dorsal skin expands arresting the infection in subcutaneous plane, rather than allowing it to enter the deeper tissues. Finally dorsal foot infection is not on the weight bearing area and therefore remains localized and does not spread during ambulation.

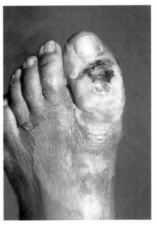

Fig. 27.1: Dorsal foot infection of left great toe

PLANTAR FOOT INFECTION (TREACHEROUS AND DEVASTATING)

Careful analysis of the history of patients with diabetic foot infection reveals, that it always begins with a delayed recognition because of lack of awareness among patients and primary care physicians, leading to delayed referral to a speciality center. Important factors responsible for this delay are:

Lack of Pain

Loss of protective sensations make a plantar abscess treacherously silent.

Out of Sight

Very few patients can carefully look at their plantars daily, for them plantar abscess is out of reach and out of sight and therefore out of mind. It is the foul smell or the stinking stained sock which brings it to notice.

Continued Ambulation

Plantar abscess is the only soft tissue infection which is on the weight bearing area. It is like a "space occupying lesion" and continued ambulation leads to proximal spread through tendon sheaths (Figs 27.2A and B). It compresses the capillary network with each loading (walking) step, causing ischemic necrosis of the soft tissue, occluding arterioles and leading to digital necrosis and gangrene.

The above mentioned factors cause delayed recognition and by the time the foot infection is recognized, it has already caused tissue damage, involvement of deeper tissues like bones and the problem is further complicated by the peculiar anatomy of the foot.

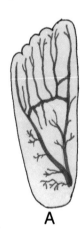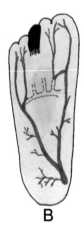

Figs 27.2A and B: **(A)** Showing normal vascular supply of plantar aspect of the foot, **(B)**Effect of central plantar abscess which works like a space occupying lesion causes occlusion of plantar arch resulting in digital necrosis

Deep Plantar Compartments (Spaces)

They are divided into medial, central and lateral compartments. When the infection is localized in one of these compartments the structures of the compartment like tendon sheaths and muscle fascia favour the proximal spread of infection. As the rigid fascial and bony structures bind these compartments, edema associated with acute infection may rapidly elevate compartment pressures, causing ischemic necrosis of the confined tissues. Finally the barriers get broken and infection spreads from one compartment to another through perforation of the intermuscular septa (Fig. 27.3).

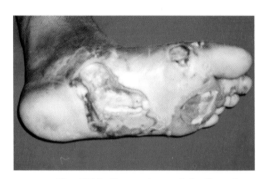

Fig. 27.3: Deep plantar infection of medial and central compartments

Foot has abundant white tissues like plantar aponeurosis, plantar fascia, tendons, ligaments, muscles sheaths, and fibrofatty subcutaneous tissue which are relatively less vascular and can neither resist infection nor withstand ischemia for too long, resulting in their necrosis. Careful assessment of foot infection is extremely important to determine the need for incision, debridement, and other surgical interventions.

Altered Host Response

Once the intact skin gets ulcerated, it paves way for the microorganisms, which release bacterial toxin and incite a host response, the wound is then defined to be infected. Normal host response is in the form of five classical local signs of inflammation due to hyperemia and inflammatory exudate. They are Heat (warmth), Redness (Erythema), Tenderness (Pain), Swelling and Loss of Function. In diabetics, two of these five signs namely tenderness (pain) and loss of function are absent because of the underlying neuropathy. As there is no pain, there is no loss of function, and as there is no loss of function the patient continues ambulation facilitating the spread of infection. In addition, diabetics have abnormatities in host defence mechanisms, especially defects in neutrophil function. The effective neutrophil antimicrobial action depends upon several factors like chemotaxis, phagocytosis and intracellular killing of the microorganisms which are altered.

What had started as a trivial plantar infection progresses to a limb threatening one and finally to a life threatening one. It is therefore of paramount importance, that every foot infection should be pursued methodically. All wounds must be carefully inspected, palpated, and probed, imaging, microbial, and other laboratory studies may then be indicated. As all the skin wounds harbor microorganisms infection must be diagnosed clinically, rather than microbiologically.

Clinical Diagnosis

Foot infection should be suspected at the first appearance of a local foot problem (e.g. pain, swelling, erythema, sinus tract, ulceration, or crepitus). Systemic spread should be suspected with the appearance of signs and symptoms such as fever, rigors, vomiting tachycardia, confusion, malaise, and loss of appetite. Metabolic disorders like severe hyperglycemia, ketosis, renal impairment, raised liver enzymes, and hyponatremia suggest septicemia and warrant urgent surgical intervention, e.g. primary amputation, in addition to aggressive medical therapy.

BACTERIOLOGICAL DIAGNOSIS

Normally fascia restricts the infection to skin and subcutaneous fat, such an infection is defined as superficial infection. When the infection invades fascia and disrupts it to enter deeper tissues like muscle, tendon, joint or bone, the infection is defined as deep infection.

Superficial infections are usually due to a single organism (monomicrobial) while deep infections are usually polymicrobial. When a wound is infected, bacterial culture will usually assist subsequent management. In patients with diabetic foot infections of longstanding and who have already received antibiotic therapy, bacterial cultures may either show mixed flora or no growth. If there is growth, culture and sensitivity results generally help to tailor antibiotic regimens. In patients who have not received antibiotics, culture and sensitivity results are more useful. Bacterial cultures should be obtained from the

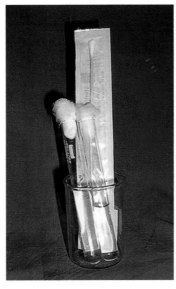

Fig. 27.4: Showing swab stick, aerobic and anaerobic culture media

base of the ulcer aseptically, or during surgery to obtain true pathogens. Specimens should be cultured for both aerobes and anaerobes (Fig. 27.4). Virulent organisms like gram-positive *Staphylococcus aureus, B hemolytic streptococci,* gram-negative organisms like *Pseudomonas aeruginosa, Klebsiella, Escherichia coli,* anaerobes like *Clostridium.* Antibiotic resistant organisms, e.g. *methicillin resistant staphylococcus aureus* (MRSA), are frequently seen in patients who have received antibiotic therapy and are usually acquired during previous hospitalization.

BONE INVOLVEMENT

Plain radiographs of the foot in anteroposterior, oblique, and lateral views (Figs 27.5 to 27.7) are essential for the diagnosis of
- Foreign body
- Gas in the soft tissue
- Osteomyelitis
- Charcot neuroarthropathy (see chapter 20).

Foreign bodies should be always looked for in traumatic injuries to the foot. Metal objects like sharp pins, needles, stapler pins, nails and broken pieces of stones have been reported to be seen.

Anaerobic organisms and some gram-negative organisms, produce gas which can be seen on a plain radiograph. It signifies infection with virulent microorganisms and needs bold and wide debridement alongwith appropriate changes in the antibiotic regimen.

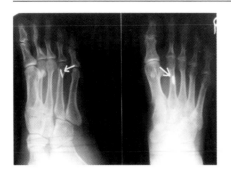

Fig. 27.5: Radiographs showing foreign body (nail)

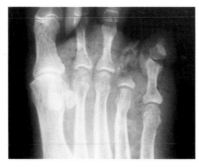

Fig. 27.6: Radiograph showing gas in the soft tissue with osteomyelitis of 4th and 5th toe phalanges

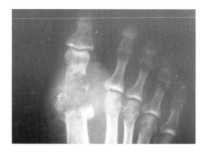

Fig. 27.7: Radiograph showing osteomyelitis of distal part of 1st metatarsal, destruction of 1st MTP joint and 1st proximal phalanx

Osteomyelitis

It generally results from contiguous spread of deep soft tissue infection through the cortex to the bone marrow. Majority of the deep longstanding foot infections are associated with osteomyelitis. Plain radiography usually shows focal osteopenia, cortical erosions or periosteal reaction in early stage and sequestration in the late stage. Radiographic changes take atleast 2 weeks to be evident. Newer techniques like bone scan, computerized tomography scan (CT) (Fig. 27.8), positron emission tomography (PET), magnetic resonance imaging (MRI) are being evaluated of which MRI is said to be more sensitive and specific. A simple clinical test is probing to bone. A sterile metal probe is inserted into the ulcer, if it penetrates to the bone, it almost confirms the diagnosis of osteomyelitis (see Fig. 23.2, chapter 23). Chronic discharging sinus or sausage like appearance of the toe are clinical markers of osteomyelitis. Definitive diagnosis requires obtaining bone biopsy for microbial culture and histopathology.

LABORATORY INVESTIGATIONS

Following investigations need to be done.
- *Complete blood counts:* Total leukocyte count is raised with a drop in hemoglobin values.
- *Erythrocyte sedimentation rate:* Raised, often above 100 mm at the end of 1st hour, in severe infections.
- *Liver enzymes:* Raised in patients with systemic toxicity.

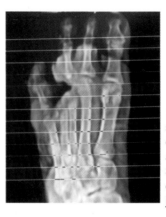

Fig. 27.8: CT scan left foot showing osteolytic destruction of 5th MTP joint, partial 4th ray amputation and destruction of 3rd MTP joint with early osteolytic changes in 2nd MTP joint

- *Renal parameters :* Serum creatinine and blood urea nitrogen are often raised in patients with septicemia.
- *Serum proteins:* Hypoalbuminemia is usually seen in longstanding foot infection.
- *Serum electrolytes:* Hyponatremia is often seen in patients with systemic toxicity.
- *Glycemic control:* Plasma glucose values are usually raised with or without ketonuria. HbA$_1$c values are raised.

SYSTEMIC EVALUATION

Longstanding diabetic foot infection leads to debility and malnutrition. The patient is often required to undergo repeated surgeries requiring anesthesia. It is therefore extremely important to assess and monitor the nutritional, cardiovascular and renal status of such patients and should receive appropriate treatment.

28 Non-Limb Threatening Infection

Caution: One thing can lead to another

Non-limb threatening infections are either superficial or if deep, they are restricted to distal part of the foot and are not associated with any significant systemic toxicity. Superficial and deep infections of toes, web space infection, dorsal foot infection, and superficial infection of the heel pad are some of the examples of non-limb threatening infections. It has to be however realized that, every non-limb threatening infection has a potential to progress to limb threatening and even life threatening infection if not arrested in time. There is no trivial lesion of the foot, every foot lesion in diabetics is vulnerable and needs to be treated aggressively.

TOE INFECTION

Infection of toe is extremely common in diabetics because of recurrent ulcerations, susceptibility to trauma, and pre-existing deformities. A deep seated infection is usually associated with erythema and cellulitis with a conspicuous absence of pain. If the infection is chronic, it invariably leads to osteomyelitis of phalanges with resultant swelling and erythema giving the toe a sausage like appearance (Fig. 28.1). The plantar aspect of the toes can get ulcerated from areas of increased plantar pressure like from tips of toes and the ball of the great toe. Laterally, they get ulcerated from injuries from the nails of adjacent toes, toe rings and ill-fitting shoes, and dorsally from physi-cal trauma and infected bunion at interphalangeal joints. Deep seated infections in toes can progress to involve MTP joints and can enter deep plantar spaces if not arrested in time, creating a limb threatening situation.

WEB SPACE INFECTION

It is particularly hazardous, because it may occur without pre-existing deformity and go unrecognized both by the patient and the physician because of the peculiar position. It may occur because of poor foot hygiene, moist environment, and mycotic infections leading to macerated whitish ulceration, which gets secondarily infected by microorganisms (Figs 28.2 and 28.3). Web space infections are particularly dangerous because of the proximity of digital arteries, which can get obliterated readily as a result. Besides, it can easily travel to the deeper structures of the foot by way of the lumbrical tendons.

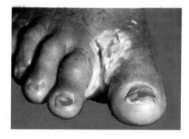

Fig. 28.2: 1st webspace infection

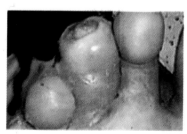

Fig. 28.1: 3rd toe showing sausage like appearance, a characteristic of osteo-myelitis

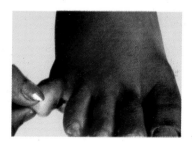

Fig. 28.3: 4th webspace infection with cellulitis

DORSAL FOOT INFECTION

The dorsum of the foot gets ulcerated usually because of extrinsic trauma. Eventhough painless, it receives prompt attention because it is easily seen. Characteristic of dorsal foot infection is marked cellulitis (Fig. 28.4).

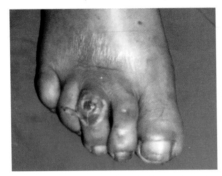

Fig. 28.4: Dorsal foot infection, secondary to ulcerated bunion 3rd toe with cellulitis

PLANTAR FOOT INFECTION

As long as the plantar foot infection is superficial, it is not limb threatening. Superficial infection of plantar ulcer, plantar wounds, and superficial infection in the heel pad are some of the examples (Figs 28.5A and B). Superficial plantar foot infections are however, noto-

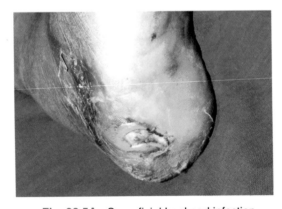

Fig. 28.5A: Superficial heel pad infection

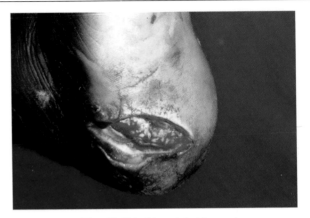

Fig. 28.5B: After debridement

rious and progress to deep plantar spaces unless aggressively managed.

Table 28.1: Indications of worsening infection	
Signs and symptons	Drainage ↑
	Erythema ↑
	Temperature ↑
	Swelling ↑
	Foul smell ↑
	Lymphangitis
	Lymphadenopathy
	Gangrene
Laboratory tests	Total leukocyte count ↑
	Erythrocyte sedimentation rate ↑
	Plasma glucose and HbA$_1$c ↑
Radiological investigations (X-ray foot)	Gas in the soft tissue
	Osteomyelitis

Trivial lesions of foot need to be aggressively treated as the clinical course can rapidly worsen from what appeared trivial just the other day, to one that now is suddenly limb or even life threatening.

29 Management of Non-Limb Threatening Infection

Rein it in well before it gallops

Majority of superficial infections (confined to skin and subcutaneous fat) are managed on an out patient basis. However, some deep infections like those of the toe, webspace, etc., need hospitalization. The principles of management are as follows:

- Glycemic control
- Antimicrobial (antibiotic) therapy
- Surgical debridement
- Care after debridement
- Prevention of recurrence

GLYCEMIC CONTROL

It is essential to achieve a good glycemic control for better infection management and healing of the wound. It is therefore advisable to switch the patients on to intensified subcutaneous insulin therapy with or without oral antidiabetic agents.

ANTIMICROBIAL (ANTIBIOTIC) THERAPY

Most of the superficial infections are monomicrobial and can be treated effectively with oral antibiotics.

Table 29.1: Commonly used oral antibiotic regimens		
Ciprofloxacin	500 mg	qid
Ofloxacin	400 mg	bid
Cephalexin	500 mg	qid
Ampicillin + Cloxacillin	250 mg + 250 mg	qid
Cefuroxime	500 mg	bid

The choice depends upon the individual's experience or culture and sensitivity report. Duration of the therapy is usually two weeks however, in deep infections, which are often polymicrobial, intravenous antibiotics for the first five days are preferred, followed by oral antibiotics for two weeks.

Table 29.2: Commonly used antibiotic regimen (intravenous)		
Cefuroxime	750 mg	bid
+ Metronidazole	500 mg	tid
Ciprofloxacin	200 mg	bid
Or		
Ofloxacin	400 mg	od
+ Metronidazole	500 mg	tid
Ceftazidime	1000 mg	bid
+ Metronidazole	500 mg	tid
Ampicillin	500 mg	qid
+ Amikacin	500 mg	tid

SURGICAL DEBRIDEMENT

Principles of Surgical Debridement

- Convert a chronic wound to an acute wound.
- Remove dead tissues like eschar (full thickness dead skin), necrotic tissue, any foreign body and the surrounding callus.
- Obtain bacterial cultures from the base of the wound.

Surgical debridement is carried out in the out-patient clinic or at the bedside. No anesthesia is usually required as the neuropathic feet are sufficiently anesthetic (insensate). Debridement is best carried out mechanically, using instruments, rather than with enzymatic or chemical agents. A scalpel, scissors and forceps are used to remove callus, necrotic tissue, eschar, etc. (Figs 29.1A to 29.1C).

Deep infections need surgical debridement in an operation theatre, under a local or a regional block anesthesia. It is necessary to carry out a thorough debridement in order to drain the pus, remove the dead and necrotic tissue. Most of the toe infections associated with osteomyelitis need toe disarticulation.

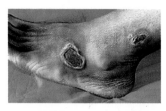

Fig. 29.1A: Eschar on dorsum and lower part of left leg

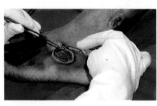

Fig. 29.1B: Eschar being removed

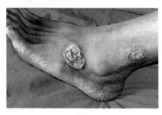

Fig. 29.1C: After removal of eschar

In great toe infections a more conservative approach is followed so as to retain as much of the great toe as possible.

CARE AFTER SURGICAL DEBRIDEMENT

The patients should be instructed to avoid weight bearing on the affected foot. The wound should be regularly cleaned with normal saline and dressed. Some debridement is often needed at intervals until the wound shows a healthy granulation tissue. Most of the superficial infections heal by primary intention, however deep infections often require secondary suturing or split skin grafting.

PREVENTION OF RECURRENCE

The patient should be educated regarding proper footcare, use of preventive footwear and explained as to how the wound had occurred and how to prevent it in future.

Case Study (29.A)

This 66 years old male with type 2 DM of 8 years, presented with swelling over the right foot dorsum and injury in the 1st web space. The patient had reported immediately after noticing the swelling. On examination there was swelling and erythema over the dorsum with purulent discharge from the wound. Debridement was carried out and the patient was

managed ambulatory on oral antibiotics. Cellulitis regressed over the period and in 4 weeks the wound completely healed (Figs 29.2A to C).

Early reporting by the patient prevented the infection from spreading to the deeper tissues.

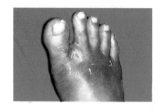

Fig. 29.2A: 1st webspace infection right foot with cellulitis

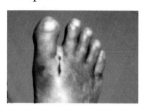

Fig. 29.2B: After debridement

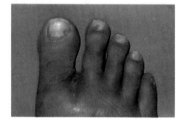

Fig. 29.2C: Wound healed

Case Study (29.B)

This 65 years old male with type 2 DM of 2 years duration presented within 5 days of noticing redness and swelling over the right foot dorsum. On examination, he had a localized abscess on the dorsolateral aspect also extending into the plantar aspect of the right foot. The cause of injury could not be ascertained. He underwent surgical debridement with the removal of necrotic material and was managed ambulatory on oral antibiotics and insulin injections. The wound healed with primary intention in six weeks (Figs 29.3 A to C).

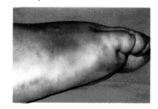

Fig. 29.3A: Localized abscess over dorsolateral part right foot

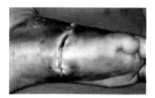

Fig. 29.3B: After incision and debridement

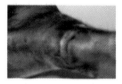

Fig. 29.3C: Wound healed

If the patient had not reported this early, the infection could have extended into the lateral compartment and progressed to a limb threatening stage.

Case Study (29.C)

This 58 years old female with type 2 DM of 8 years, presented with non-healing wound on the right 2nd toe and 2nd web space, since 8 weeks. The cause of wound was not known. On examination, she had neuropathic feet with a normal ABI and swelling of 2nd and 3rd toes of the right foot (Fig. 29.4A). There was a sinus on the tip of the 2nd toe, discharging purulent material. X-ray of the foot revealed osteomyelitis of the two distal phalanges of the 2nd toe.

The patient was hospitalized, switched on to insulin and I/V antibiotics. **Disarticulation of the 2nd and 3rd toes** at MTP joints was carried out alongwith the removal of necrotic tissue, keeping the wound open (open amputation) and preserving some viable skin of the 2nd toe (Fig. 29.4B). The third toe was disarticulated as it was also found to be infected. Six weeks later, patient's wound was sutured using the redundant skin and six months later, the patient had developed hallux valgus deformity of the right great toe, as it had lost support of 2 lateral toes (Fig. 29.4C).

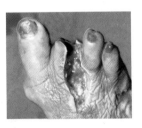

Fig. 29.4A: Infected 2nd and 3rd toe with 2nd webspace infection right foot

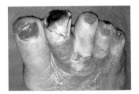

Fig. 29.4B: After disarticulation of 2nd and 3rd toes at MTP joints

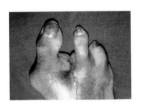

Fig. 29.4C: Wound closed with sutures using the redundant skin, note hallux valgus

Such deep infections (Grade 3 of Wagner's) of toes have a potential to destroy MTP joints and enter the deep plantar compartments.

Case Study (29.D)

This 49 years old male, with type 2 DM of 8 years duration, was referred for non-healing ulcer on the left heel. History revealed that he had sustained an injury following which, he developed swelling over the heel. He had undergone surgical debridement elsewhere however, the wound was not healing despite dressings and antibiotics for 2 months. The wound was healthy with red granulation tissue, his X-ray did not reveal osteomyelitis and duplex Doppler study revealed a patent posterior tibial artery. The cause of non-healing wound was continued ambulation, as he was a fruit vendor. He was advised crutches and was reviewed fortnightly. The ulcer gradually healed with complete epithelialization (Figs 29.5A to C).

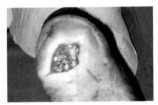

Fig. 29.5A: Non-healing ulcer over left heel

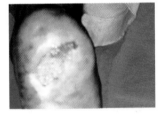

Fig. 29.5B: Healing heel ulcer

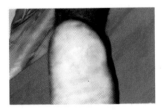

Fig. 29.5C: Heel ulcer healed with epithelialization

Heel ulcers are difficult to heal. Once the heel pad gets infected, the situation can worsen to a limb threatening one, especially, if the calcaneus is infected. Non-weight bearing is extremely important when the ulcer is active.

30 Limb Threatening Infection

Danger: Limb today, Life tomorrow

Limb threatening infection is a medicosurgical emergency. Patients have evidence of systemic toxicity due to longstanding infection. Characteristic limb threatening infections are dorsal foot infections with cellulitis (phlegmon), plantar compartment infections, and deep infections of the heel pad. Limb threatening situation indicates that it is certainly going to require nothing less than a leg amputation, unless aggressively managed.

DORSAL FOOT INFECTION WITH CELLULITIS

The clinical presentation is in the form of extensive cellulitis. Infection in dorsum of the foot spreads via lymphatics. In diabetics with neuropathy such extensive cellulitis is not associated with pain and tenderness, thus allowing ambulation and dependent position causing further spread of infection. A person with normal sensations would automatically rest and elevate the foot because of pain. Dorsal compartment of the foot has all extensor muscle tendons which are not encased in sheaths but lie in loose areolar tissue. Thin superficial fascia which covers these extensor tendons is continuous with the extensor retinaculum of the ankle and infection can spread along these

tendons proximally from foot into the leg. Such a swollen and infected foot dampens the arterial blood flow and skin over dorsum of the foot can get easily necrosed due to infective occlusions of small vessels in the skin (Figs 30.1 to 30.3).

INFECTIONS IN PLANTAR COMPARTMENTS

There are three plantar compartments namely lateral, central, and medial.

Infection in the Lateral Compartment

The lateral compartment is bound by the fifth metatarsal dorsally, an inter muscular septum medially, and the edge of the plantar aponeurosis laterally. It contains the abductor and short flexor muscles of the fifth toe. Infection enters this compartment from infected bunionette of the 5th toe, web space infection between 4th and 5th toes, shoe bite, direct penetrating injuries, digital infection of the little toe, or deep infection in the plantar ulcer over 5th metatarsal head. It clinically manifests as swelling and erythema on the lateral side of the forefoot, with or without necrosis of the fifth toe (Fig. 30.4). Dorsum of the foot is often swollen, but in the absence of pain,

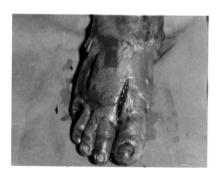
Fig. 30.1: Severe dorsal foot infection right foot, with cellulitis

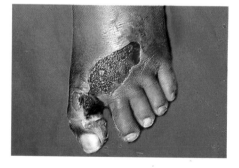
Fig. 30.2: Dorsal foot infection with gangrene left great toe

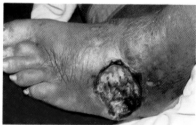
Fig. 30.3: Dorsal foot infection left foot

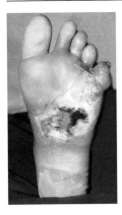

Fig. 30.4: Lateral compartment infection with necrosis left 5th toe

the patient is relatively asymptomatic. If not managed in time, such infection can progress into the central compartment which can prove devastating.

Infection in Medial Compartment

The medial compartment is bound by the first metatarsal dorsally, an extension of the plantar aponeurosis medially, and intermuscular septum laterally. It contains the abductor and flexor muscles of the great toe. Infection enters the medial compartment through erosion of the MTP joint of the great toe, or from physical trauma such as penetrating injuries, shoe bite, nail infection, or web space infection between first and second toes. Once infection is established, the foot is swollen medially, the medial arch disappears, plantar skin is swollen, and erythematous with or without, edema over dorsum of the foot. Infection can progress proximally through the tendon of flexor hallucis longus or can enter the central plantar compartment, by disruption of the intermuscular septum (Fig. 30.5).

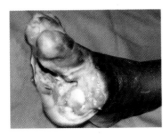

Fig. 30.5: Medial compartment infection has spread proximally despite right great toe disarticulation

Infection in Central Plantar Compartment

The central compartment is bound by the plantar aponeurosis inferiorly, intermuscular septa medially and laterally, and tarsals and metatarsals dorsally. It contains lumbricals, flexors to the digits, adductor

hallucis, and posterior tibial and peroneal tendons. Infection in the central plantar compartment is most devastating. It enters from web spaces, toe infections, penetrating injuries or from plantar ulcers over the metatarsal heads. The plantar digital arteries of the second, third and fourth toes arise from the plantar arch. Thrombotic obliteration of the plantar arch can lead to digital necrosis of these toes particularly of the third toe (Fig. 30.6). Once the infection is established, the longitudinal arch and the plantar skin creases disappear. There is swelling and erythema of the sole and edema over dorsum of the foot.

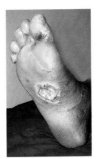

Fig. 30.6: Central compartment infection right foot, note destruction of 3rd toe

All the plantar compartment infections are on the weight bearing areas and ambulation in absence of pain can lead to pressure necrosis of the soft tissue, capillaries, and milking action facilitating further spread proximally. Along the flexor tendon, the infection can progress along the muscle tendons beyond ankle into the leg.

DEEP INFECTION IN THE HEEL PAD

The heel is a vulnerable area and being the most proximal part of the foot, any deep seated infection can be a limb threatening situation. The heel pad is abundant in fatty tissue and is short of red muscle mass. Infection leads to fat necrosis and as there is no intervening red muscle mass, it can easily spread into calcaneus (Fig. 30.7). The heel is infected either as an

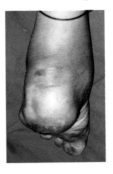

Fig. 30.7: Heel pad infection

extension of infection from mid foot or through pene-trating injuries, plantar ulcers, fissures, or through decubitus ulcer.

In limb threatening infection, systemic toxicity is usually evident in the form of fever, malaise, loss of appetite, vomiting, and pallor. The glycemic control is invariably poor and the patient can even present with ketoacidosis. Such patients if not managed promptly, a life threatening situation can soon arise.

31 Management of Limb Threatening Infection

Body moans for the losing limb

Limb threatening infection is a deep seated infection of the various plantar compartments, deep infections of the heel, and dorsum of the foot. There is often a suppurative process with involvement of deeper tissues like muscles, tendons and bones with areas of necrosis. There is evidence of systemic toxicity.

The diabetic foot with a deep seated infection is very deceptive and it is not always possible to judge the extent of infection and tissue damage by just a local examination. It is best revealed during radical surgical debridement. It is not uncommon that the definitive surgery planned has to be revised, in favor of a more radical excision or even a proximal or major amputation. It is our practice to call a responsible relative of the patient inside the theatre, to be shown the severity of the lesion and to obtain an appropriate consent for a more radical surgery.

Most of the times, these patients have longstanding infected lesions and are moribund, debilitated and toxic, hence it is a prerequisite to thoroughly evaluate the patient clinically and biochemically. The cardiac, renal, and nutritional status needs to be studied and appropriate measures taken so that the patient can withstand for anesthesia.

PRINCIPLES OF MANAGEMENT

- Supportive treatment
- Glycemic control
- Antibiotic therapy
- Surgical debridement
- Postoperative care of the wound
- Closure of the wound
- Prevention of recurrence

Supportive Treatment

It includes correction of hydration, electrolyte imbalance, anemia (blood transfusion), hypoalbuminemia, ensuring an adequate calorie intake (oral or parenteral) and stabilization of blood pressure.

Glycemic Control

These patients have invariably a poor glycemic control as evident by a raised plasma glucose and HbA_1c values, ketonuria or even ketoacidosis. It is not uncommon to see the anesthetist or even the surgeon refusing to operate because of a poorly controlled diabetes. The physician finds it difficult to achieve a good glycemic control in presence of severe infection. The delay in surgery often leads to more proximal spread of infection. At our centre we treat these patients with intravenous infusion of insulin and post the patient for radical debridement within 48 hours.

Table 31.1: Intravenous insulin regimen *(100 units of regular human insulin in 100 ml bottle of normal saline (1 unit / 1ml) is given intravenous. The dose is titrated as per the prevailing plasma glucose)*

Plasma glucose mg %	(mmol)	Insulin infusion (units/h)
< 50	(2.7)	Turn off infusion for 15 min administer 25 ml 25% glucose
50-70	(2.7-3.88)	0.5
70-120	(3.88-6.6)	1
120-180	(6.6-10)	1.5
180-280	(10-15.55)	2
280-360	(15.55-20)	4
> 360	(20)	5 + Bolus 10 units intravenous

(Plasma glucose should be estimated every 2 hours)

Insulin resistance is present when the patient is harboring a severe foot infection and the insulin requirement is reduced dramatically after a radical surgical debridement. In fact reduction in insulin requirement with a stable plasma glucose values are indirect indicators that the infection is getting controlled. The patient should be switched over to intensified subcutaneous insulin (multiple injections) postoperatively after oral feeding is resumed.

ANTIBIOTIC THERAPY

The deep infection in diabetic foot is invariably polymicrobial. It is essential to obtain a fresh wound culture and another sample is obtained during the surgery. It is always preferable to administer intravenous antibiotics. The choice of antibiotics depends upon the individual experience, severity of infection, presence of crepitus, or gas in the soft tissue, and evidence of systemic toxicity.

An antibiotic regimen should almost always include an agent active against staphylococci, streptococci, and gram-negative organisms. When culture and sensitivity reports are available, an antibiotic regimen can be revised, narrowed, and tailored accordingly. The duration of therapy depends upon the severity of infection and the response of the patient. In localized infections, intravenous antibiotics are given for one week followed by oral antibiotics for atleast two weeks. In severe infections, intravenous antibiotics are often required for two weeks followed by oral antibiotics for another two to four weeks. In patients with osteomyelitis, the duration of antibiotic therapy may be prolonged, however in most of the patients it is preferable to remove the infected bone during debridement, thereby facilitating a quicker healing of the wound.

Table 31.2: Commonly used antibiotic regimen (intravenous)		
Cefuroxime	750 mg	bid
+ Metronidazole	500 mg	tid
Ciprofloxacin	200 mg	bid
Or		
Ofloxacin	400 mg	od
+ Metronidazole	500 mg	tid
Ceftazidime	1 g	bid
+ Metronidazole	500 mg	tid
Ampicillin	500 mg	qid
+ Amikacin	500 mg	tid
Sulbactum/Cefoperazone (1:1)	1 to 2 g	bid

(Note : There are newer antibiotics and combinations available, treating footcare team should make their own choice depending on their experience and the bacteriological results)

SURGICAL DEBRIDEMENT

Patients with deep seated infection need radical surgical debridement. Infected foot is one area of surgery where "pinhole surgery" does not work. All patients with a deep seated infection should undergo debridement in an operation theatre; temptation to operate by the bedside should be avoided. Most of the distal foot infections can be operated upon under a local anesthesia such as an ankle block, others need either spinal or general anesthesia.

Table 31.3: Principles of surgical debridement	
Aim	Convert chronic wound into an acute one Convert infected wound into a surgical one
Incision	Single or multiple, long and deep Preferably on non-weight bearing areas
Debridement	Should open all infected deeper compartments. Should drain pus Should remove all that is necrotic and dead (skin, muscles, soft tissue, tendons and bones) Should conserve healthy tissue

Early surgical intervention with a thorough debridement helps in reducing the duration of antibiotic therapy, decreases the need for major amputations, conserves some of the viable tissue which is compromised and helps in evaluating the extent of the tissue damage. All deep compartments involved by infection must be opened, pus pockets drained and all the necrotic dead tissue including skin, muscles, tendons, aponeurosis, ligaments, and even the bones removed, conserving the healthy tissue. Bacterial cultures should be obtained from deeper areas, infected tissues and excised bones. Thorough surgical debridement should be so efficiently carried out (Figs 31.1 to 31.6), that no further debridement is required, although few patients do require a repeat debridement after a week or so.

The patient starts improving after debridement surgery; his appetite improves, the smile returns on the face, and signs of systemic toxicity start reducing, a sense of well being is apparent and the insulin requirement is reduced.

Therapy of Osteomyelitis

Osteomyelitis is a common feature of deep tissue infection of the foot. In majority of the cases, the treatment of choice is complete resection of the infected bone

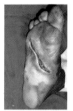

Fig. 31.1: Linear bold incision for debridement avoiding weight bearing areas

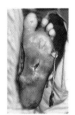

Fig. 31.2: Multiple incisions, one on midplantar area another on medial border of the foot avoiding weight bearing areas, disarticulation of 5th toe has further facilitated drainage and removal of necrotic tissue

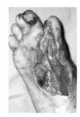

Fig. 31.3: Debridement for infected plantar ulcer on the great toe with extension in medial plantar compartment

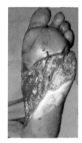

Fig. 31.4: Bold radical debridement for deep plantar compartment infection, extending from lateral to central and medial compartment with 5th toe disarticulation

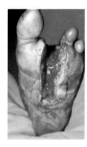

Fig. 31.5: Wedge resection for central compartment infection with 2nd and 3rd ray amputations

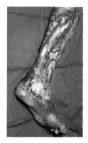

Fig. 31.6: Bold radical fasciotomy for infection spreading into the leg

(e.g. phalanges and metatarsals) (Figs 31.7A to 31.8C). Osteomyelitis of calcaneus is a difficult surgical problem. It is often associated with the heel pad infection. Removal of infected tissue along with scooping of the infected bone should be tried. This therapy has to be associated with strict non-weight bearing and prolonged intravenous antibiotics. In patients with destruction of calcaneus, salvaging the foot is extremely difficult. Removal of calcaneus or Syme's amputation are not feasible, as the heel pad is invari-

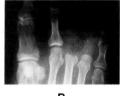 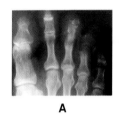 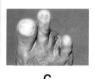

A   B   C

Figs 31.8A to C: (A) Radiograph showing osteomyelitis of phalanges of 3rd and 4th toes, (B) Radiograph showing disarticulation at 3rd and 4th MTP joints, (C) Wound healed completely after suturing of the redundant skin

ably badly infected. Such patients often need a leg amputation.

Some studies have shown however, that diabetic foot osteomyelitis can be arrested and in some, even cured with the higher doses of antibiotics given for prolonged period ranging between 2 to 6 months. We have a limited experience in treating osteomyelitis in the diabetic foot conservatively by using prolonged antibiotics and strict non weight bearing (Figs 31.9A to 31.10C)

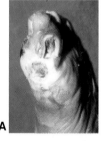

A

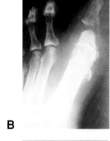

B

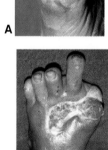

C

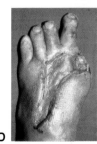

D

Figs 31.7A to D: (A) Infected great toe with necrotic ulcer on medial border of great toe and 1st MTP joint, (B) Radiograph showing osteomyelitis with destruction of 1st IP joint, (C) Disarticulation performed at 1st MTP joints (D) Skin defect closed, by skin grafting

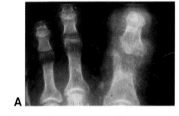

A

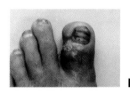

B

Fig. 31.9A and B: (A) Radiograph showing osteomyelitis with destruction of 1st IP joint left foot, (B) Discharging sinus on lateral aspect of left great toe, completely healed with prolonged antibiotics and strict non-weight bearing without surgery

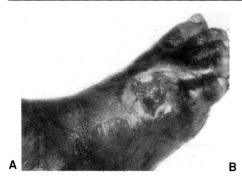
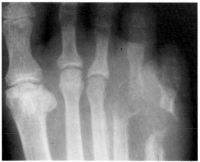
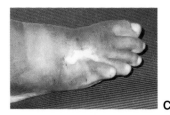

Fig. 31.10A to C: **(A)** 4th web space infection extending into dorsum of the foot, **(B)** Radiograph of right foot shows osteolytic destruction of 4th and 5th MTP joints, **(C)** Wound completely healed with prolonged antibiotics and immobilization without surgery

Hyperbaric Oxygen Therapy (HBO)

It is an adjunct to current medical and surgical treatment of advanced foot lesions like Wagner's grades 3 to 5. It is rendered in specially designed chambers and is usually given twice a day for about 90 to 120 minutes. HBO therapy increases tissue oxygen tension which is essential for wound healing. It increases fibroblast proliferation, angiogenesis, collagen deposition and enhances bacterial killing. It is expensive and is not readily available. Therefore its use is restricted to treat severe foot infections that have not responded to other treatment.

Postoperative Care of the Wound

Rest to the part (strict non-weight bearing) from day one is the most important aspect (Fig. 31.11). It is not uncommon to see a diabetic patient walking after debridement surgery, in the hospital wards. Ambulation without crutches should be strictly discouraged. The wound should be thoroughly irrigated with normal saline. A 20 ml syringe with 18 gauge angiocath may be used to irrigate the wound with normal saline.

Immersing the foot in lukewarm water with antiseptic solution is a common practice even today. The entire foot is immersed in a tub of water (often warm water) with antiseptic solutions (Fig. 31.12). The patient is instructed to dorsiflex and plantar flex the foot. Such a bath is given for fifteen to twenty minutes and if the attending nurse is being elsewhere, the patient often enjoys the foot bath for even an hour. Universal experience has been that water bath is harmful and should be avoided. It leads to overhydration causing maceration of the toe webs, nail folds, and heel tissue and promotes spread of the infection. In the presence of exposed bones, joints or deep sinuses, water bath can be detrimental. Such a water bath is therefore best avoided. Regular bedside debridement is necessary for removal of fresh necrotic tissues. In some patients with purulent infection, second debridement is required after a week or so, if there are signs of persistent infection or fresh areas of necrosis.

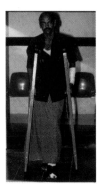

Fig. 31.11: Strict non-weight bearing from day one using crutches

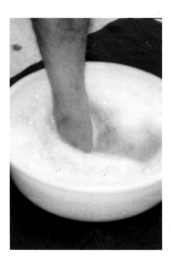

Fig. 31.12: Foot bath is often harmful and not warranted

Dressings

After cleaning the wound with normal saline, antibacterial agents are often used. We use diluted povidone iodine. I have seen surgeons emptying a whole bottle of spirit and hydrogen peroxide on wounds. Such indiscriminate use does more harm than benefit, as they are harmful to budding granulation tissue. The wound should be dressed more frequently if there is a soakage, otherwise once daily. The dressing should be moist, as moist environment encourages wound regeneration and healing. Absorbent used to remove the exudates should be sterile and porous to allow a gaseous exchange thereby protecting the wound from a secondary infection. Dressings get adherent and can cause harm; such adherent dressings should be pre-soaked in normal saline before removal. The surgeon should have a look at the wound on the postoperative day and then atleast every third or fourth day. Patients can get fever with chills after the dressing because of handling of the tissue, resulting in transient bacteremia. Signs of improvement are visible in a few days in the form of reduction in soakage and drainage of the pus or exudative material. Red healthy granulation tissue becomes visible after two to three weeks, the wound size is reduced, sinus tracts and cavities fill up, and in about four weeks most of the wounds are healthy. Patients who have undergone extensive debridement, skin grafting, and mid foot amputation need to be given a posterior cast so as to maintain the foot in its position of function (Fig. 31.13), to prevent deformities.

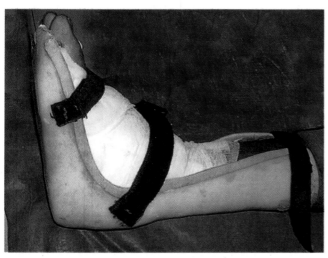

Fig. 31.13: Foot in posterior cast

Closure of the Wound

Once the wound is infection free, not discharging and is filling up with the red granulation tissue, the strategies for closure of the wound can be planned depending upon the size and site of the defect. If the initial debridement has not been associated with a significant skin loss, the wound closes by epithelization or it can be closed by loose sutures after few days of debridement. The wounds with larger defects however need closure either by suturing after undermining the edges or by split skin grafting (Figs 31.14 to 31.16).

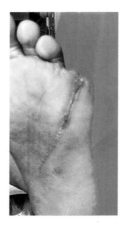

Fig. 31.14: Wound healed by epithelialization

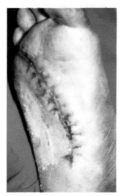

Fig. 31.15: Wound closed by secondary suturing

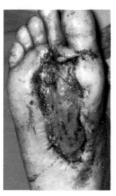

Fig. 31.16: Wound defect closed by split skin grafting

Having a plastic and reconstructive surgeon in the diabetic footcare team is of paramount importance and our diabetic footcare team is fortunate to have one. They have certain special qualities notably an immense respect for the tissues. While debriding they conserve the viable skin with an eye on the future closure of the wound. They consider every graft they put as their prestige and therefore are always concerned and like to keep a close followup of the patient. Although, they are masters in delicate aspects of cosmetic surgery, because of their training in cancer surgery, they are equally proficient in devastating surgeries like fasciotomy and radical surgical debridement of the diabetic foot.

Although many techniques of tissue transfer, local skin and muscle flaps have been described for wound closure, the commonest procedure used is the split skin graft. The most challenging area for grafting is plantar skin defect obviously because it has to tolerate the trauma of weight bearing. Conversely, the dorsal foot does not have a weight bearing surface and hence a split skin graft works best in this location. Management of deep infections in diabetic foot with foot salvage is a long drawn battle and often requires two to three months for final closure of the wound.

PREVENTION OF RECURRENCE

After successful management of an infected diabetic foot, the challenge before the diabetic footcare team is to prevent the recurrence. Infection recurs in about 20% of patients, many of whom have underlying and often undiagnosed osteomyelitis.

The patient has to be made to realize that the healed foot is never quite the same again. It needs much more meticulous care than any other insensate foot. Patient has to undertake gradual ambulation and keep the activity level to a minimum. The scar tissue is different from the normal sole in several ways.

- It is hard, non elastic and therefore does not cushion the foot as it hits the ground.
- The skin over the scar is very thin and gets traumatized easily.
- It has a poor blood supply and is thus slow to heal when injured.

The patients should wear a protective cushioned footwear regularly and should be reviewed in the clinic atleast monthly. It is gratifying to salvage the foot in a patient with limb threatening infection.

However, with infections involving deeper structures, a salvage may require some form of minor amputation, the commonest being a toe amputation. Although the goal is to salvage the foot in every limb threatening infection, there are occasions, when despite radical surgical debridement the wound fails to show improvement, so also the general condition of the patient. In such situation, the footcare team should not hesitate in revising the management strategy in favour of a more proximal foot or even a limb amputation, as any further delay can prove life threatening.

Case Study (31.A)

This 51 years old female with type 1 DM of 18 years duration, presented with fever, swelling of the left foot since 1 week, and discharging wound over the dorsum since 5 days secondary to some unknown injury. Her general physical and systemic examinations were normal except that she was febrile. There were no signs of ketoacidosis. Examination of the left foot showed marked cellulitis over the dorsum with a blister and nectrotic skin on the dorsolateral aspect extending into the 4th webspace (Fig. 31.17A). On pressing, there was purulent discharge from the wound. She had evidence of neuropathy with normal ABI.

She was hospitalized and switched on to I/V broad spectrum antibiotics, metronidazole and intensified insulin therapy. Her investigations revealed Hb 12gms%, TLC 12,200/cu.mm, ESR 68 mm/1st hr, S. creatinine 0.8 mg/dL, plasma glucose of 312 mg% and HbA$_1$c 8.9%. There was no ketonuria. The X-ray of the foot did not reveal any evidence of osteomyelitis or gas in the soft tissues.

She was posted for radical debridement surgery, where the necrotic and infected tissues were removed (Fig. 31.17B). The patient was discharged after five days of hospitalization and was followed up regularly. In 4 weeks' time, the wound was covered with a granulation tissue, except for a small area of slough. As the patient was unwilling for skin grafting, it took a longer duration and the wound healed with a scar (Fig. 31.17C)

This is an excellent example of limb threatening dorsal foot infection, where the foot could be salvaged because of timely intervention. The characteristics of dorsal foot infection are marked cellulitis, rapid necrosis of skin and its propensity to spread

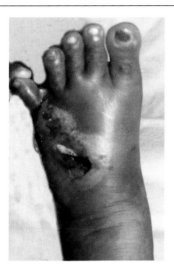

Fig. 31.17A: 4th webspace infection extending into the dorsum of left foot, necrotic skin, ruptured purulent bulla

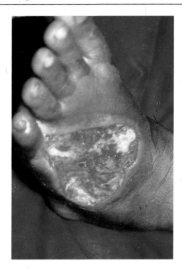

Fig. 31.17B: After radical surgical debridement

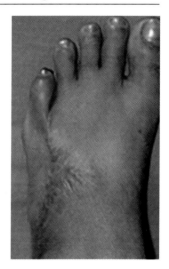

Fig. 31.17C: Wound healed with scarring

proximally into the leg along the superficial fascia covering the extensor tendons.

Case Study (31.B)

This 52 years old male with type 2 DM of 6 years, a police constable by profession, non-smoker, presented with a non-healing wound on the left foot, swelling, and fever. He sustained this wound secondary to an unknown injury, following which he noticed gradually increasing swelling and discoloration. On examination, he was toxic, febrile, pulse rate was 124/min with BP of 130/80 mmHg. Systemic examination was normal. Local examination revealed a swollen left foot, blisters on the dorsum of the foot with purulent discharge, the great toe and medial aspect of the forefoot skin was gangrenous (Fig. 31.18A). On palpation, there was malodorus purulent discharge from the margins of the gangrenous skin. The plantar skin was swollen and erythematous, especially medially. One of the blisters on the dorsum of the foot

extended upto the medial malleolus with surrounding erythema. The patient had a neuropathic foot with a normal ABI and the X-ray foot did not reveal any osteomyelitis. His Hb was 9.2 gm%, TLC was 16,800/cu.mm, ESR 110 mm/1st hr, renal, hepatic and cardiac parameters were normal.

The clinical impression was an advanced deep tissue infection of the left foot involving both the dorsal and plantar aspects with extensive destruction of the soft tissues but preserved heel pad. He was hospitalized, switched on to intravenous antibiotics, and multiple injections of insulin and mid foot amputation was planned with the exact level to be decided intraoperatively. The patient eventually required a **mid tarsal amputation** (Fig. 31.18B). The wound was left open. He received 2 units of blood, intravenous antibiotics for 2 weeks, and was discharged after 3 weeks. The wound healed completely after 2 months of discharge from the hospital (Fig. 31.18C). The patient was given special shoes and was advised to change the job nature to a sedentary one.

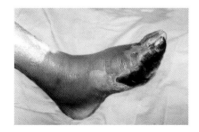

Fig. 31.18A: Swollen infected left foot, gangrene great toe, purulent bulla

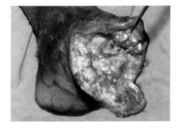

Fig. 31.18B: Midtarsal amputation, intraoperative picture

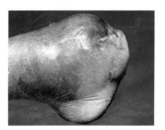

Fig. 31.18C: The stump healed completely

Case Study (31.C)

This 58 years old male with type 2 DM of 6 years, presented with blackening of the right great toe with swelling and discharging wound on the dorsum of the right foot since two and half months. History revealed that the wound had resulted after a silencer pipe injury for which the patient had received antibiotics, dressings and surgical debridement but the wound continued to deteriorate.

On examination, the patient had a neuropathic foot, normal ABI, gangrene of the right great toe, and debrided wound on the dorsum revealed slough, malodorous discharge and underlying red granulation tissue. There were marks of vitiligo on the foot (Fig. 31.19A). The X-ray of the foot revealed periosteal reaction of the phalanges and destruction of the 1st MTP joint.

The patient was hospitalized, switched on to intravenous antibiotics, and multiple injections of insulin. He was then subjected to a surgical debridement and **1st ray amputation,** which involved removal of the great toe and proximal part of the 1st metatarsal alongwith slough and necrotic tissue. The wound was left open (Fig. 31.19B). After 5 days of intravenous antibiotics, the patient was discharged from the hospital and switched on to oral antibiotics. The wound healed with primary intention in 2 months (Fig. 31.19C).

Although, it started as a thermal injury, the ulceration got secondarily infected leading to septic arteritis and digital necrosis. The deep tissue involvement occurred because of continued ambulation in presence of poor glycemic control. The earlier surgical debridement was inadequate. Such deep tissue infection of **medial compartment** can enter central plantar compartment leading to further destruction of the foot.

Case Study (31.D)

This 66 years old female with type 2 DM of 18 years duration and hypertension since 8 years presented with fever and swelling of the left foot since 2 weeks. Her general physical examination was normal except for BP of 160/100 mmHg. Her systemic examination was normal. She had neuropathic feet with a normal ABI. Her left foot was swollen on the plantar aspect with evidence of deep **central compartment infection**. The patient also had a callosity over the great toe and toe deformities. She was hospitalized, switched on to

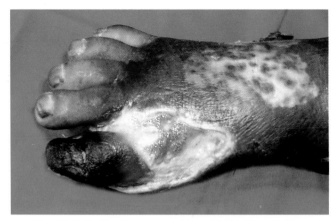
Fig. 31.19A: Gangrenous right great toe, slough in an already debrided wound

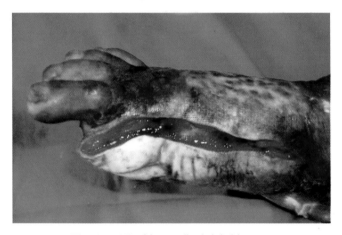
Fig. 31.19B: After radical debridement and 1st ray amputation

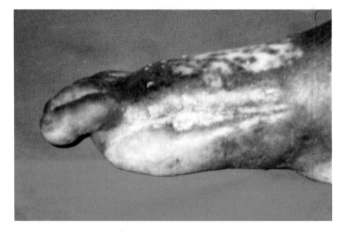
Fig. 31.19C: Wound healed

intravenous antibiotics and multiple insulin injections and subjected to extensive debridement (Fig. 31.20 A). After 4 weeks of regular dressings, the wound was closed with a split skin graft (Fig. 31.20 B). The patient

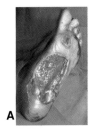
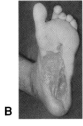

Figs 31.20A and B: **(A)** Central compartment infection left foot after debridement, note callosity 1st MTH, **(B)** Plantar defect closed by skin graft, callosity at 1st MTH removed

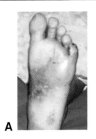
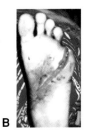
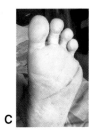

Fig. 31.21A to C: **(A)** Left lateral compartment infection after sharp injury (fishbone), necrotic 5th toe, **(B)** After radical debridement with 5th toe disarticulation, **(C)** Wound healed by epithelialization and scarring

walked with this foot for 8 long years before she died of cerebral hemorrhage but with an intact foot.

Case Study (31.E)

This 58 years old female with type 2 DM of 16 years duration, presented with swelling and redness of the left foot, ulceration of the little toe, and fever with rigors. She was being treated elsewhere with oral antidiabetics and dressings. History revealed that 3 weeks ago, she had accidentally stepped on to a fish bone which had fallen out from the overflowing dustbin. Her general physical and systemic examinations were normal. Local examination revealed an ulcer over the left 5th toe, cellulitis on the dorsum, and swelling on the lateral plantar aspect (Fig. 31.21A) with extension medially. There was pus discharge in the 4th web space on pressure over the plantar aspect. Her investigations revealed Hb 10.5 gm%, TLC 7200/cu.mm, ESR 85 mm/1st hour, S. creatinine 0.7 mg/dL, plasma glucose 242 mg% and HbA$_1$c 8.5%. She had an evidence of background retinopathy and incipient nephropathy. Her resting ECG was normal. X-ray of the foot revealed osteomyelitis of the 5th toe phalanges. A clinical diagnosis of deep seated infection of the left 5th toe and **lateral compartment** with extension into the **central compartment** was made.

She was hospitalized, switched onto IV antibiotics, intensified insulin therapy and posted for debridement. She underwent disarticulation of the 5th toe at MTP joint and through a bold incision extending from the base of the 5th MT head to medial border of the foot. The necrotic tissue and purulent material were removed (Fig. 31.21B). After 1 week, she was discharged with instructions of strict non weight bearing (use of crutches), regular dressings, insulin, and oral antibiotics. Four weeks later the plantar wound got approximated and after 2 months of surgery the wound healed completely with epithelialization leaving a scar (Fig. 31.21C).

Sharp injuries are often the cause of deep seated plantar infection. The lateral compartment infection, if not aggressively treated, breaks open into the central compartment leading to extensive destruction of the foot.

Case Study (31.F)

This 46 years old male with type 2 DM of 6 years duration, presented with swelling of the right foot. His general physical and systemic examinations were normal. He had neuropathic feet with a normal ABI. History revealed that he had sustained sharp injury to the midfoot which developed into a deep plantar infection. It had also migrated to the dorsum leading to cellulitis. He had undergone surgical debridement elsewhere which was inadequate, as is evident from the small incision on the lateral plantar aspect, and on the dorsum as evident from the necrotic tissue and slough (Fig. 31.22 A, 31.22D).

His investigations revealed Hb 8 gm%, TLC 14,000/cu.mm, ESR 92 mm/1st hr, S. Creatinine 1.4 mg/dl, HbA$_1$c of 10.2% and plasma glucose of 410 mg%. He was hospitalized, switched on to intravenous antibiotics and multiple insulin injections and was posted for debridement.

He underwent extensive debridement with removal of the necrotic tissue and slough. The extent of debridement covered the dorsolateral aspect of the foot almost entirely and also extended into the anterolateral aspect of the lower thirds of the leg. On the plantar aspect it covered the mid foot and extended upto the medial malleolus (Figs 31.22B, 31.22E). He required regular dressings for the following 3 weeks after which both, the dorsal and plantar wounds were simultaneously covered in the same sitting, with a split skin graft (Figs 31.22C, 31.22 F).

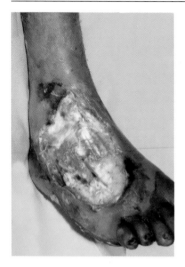

Fig. 31.22A: Inadequate
debridement, dorsal aspect

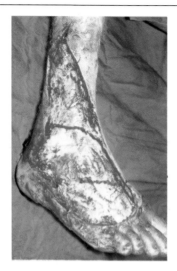

Fig. 31.22B: After radical
debridement

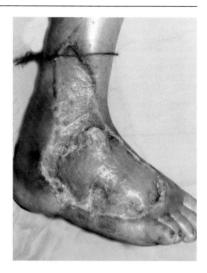

Fig. 31.22C: After skin grafting,
dorsal wound

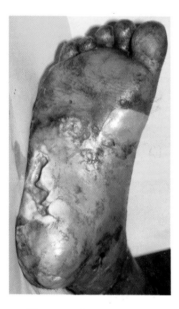

Fig. 31.22D: Inadequate
debridement, plantar aspect

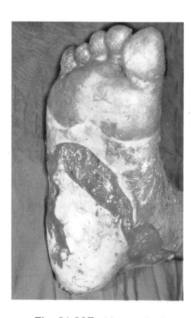

Fig. 31.22E: After radical
debridement

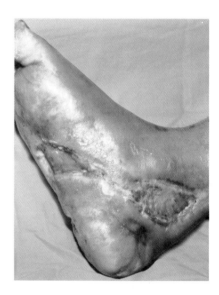

Fig. 31.22F: After skin grafting,
plantar defect

Inadequate debridement, unfortunately a common scenario and is the frequent cause of worsening of a wound as in this case. This case is an excellent example of extensive bold surgical debridement of deep infection involving both dorsal and plantar aspects of the foot, resulting in the salvage of the limb.

32 Necrotizing Fascitis

It spreads like a wild fire

In tissues adjoining infection, small vessels commonly develop thrombotic occlusion leading to necrosis of the tissue. After desloughing, draining or control of infection, normal arterioles recanalize and form granulation tissue promoting healing of the wound. However in certain mixed infections, so common in diabetic foot, virulent strains of staphylococci and streptococci liberate angiotoxic (necrotizing) substances. These angiotoxic factors like alpha-toxin of staphylococci, along with spreading factors like streptokinase and streptococcal hyaluronidase lead to a rapid extension of necrosis by digestion of fibrin barriers and intracellular ground substance. This is a severe, progressive soft tissue infection, which leads to necrosis of subcutaneous tissues down to the level of muscle fascia. Clinically, it begins with a trivial infection in foot or hand leading to rapidly advancing necrosis with erythema, swelling, and dusky discoloration of the overlying skin with hemorrhagic blisters (Figs 32.1 and 32.2). The occlusive process in the small vessels is exaggerated, more arterioles are obliterated and the original lesions get converted from trivial to ever enlarging areas of necrosis and gangrene. Creeping advancement of this process of infective obliterative angiopathy leads to devastating lesions within a couple of days. There is also evidence of systemic toxicity in the form of fever, tachycardia, and hypotension. Urgent fasciotomy, fasciectomy, and if required a major amputation needs to be carried out along with an aggressive medical treatment to prevent such a life threatening situation (Figs 32.3 A and B).

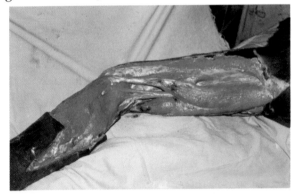

Fig. 32.3A: After extensive fasciectomy left leg, muscles and femoral vessels seen (posterior view)

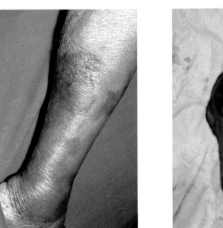

Fig. 32.1: Right leg showing erythema, swelling and dusky discoloration

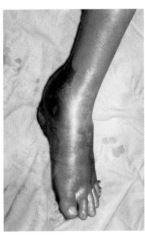

Fig. 32.2: Left foot and leg showing swelling erythema and hemorrhagic bulla

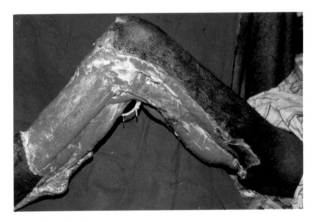

Fig. 32.3B: Lateral view after extensive fasciectomy

We recollect having done only one hip disarticulation, one knee disarticulation and one shoulder disarticulation at our centre, in the last two decades. In all these cases the indication for amputation was extensive necrotizing fascitis. One who underwent hip disarticulation succumbed, whereas the other two made an uneventful recovery.

Case Study (32.A)

This 56 years old male, an employee in university, presented in a critical situation with a history of high grade fever since 4 days, swollen right leg, breathlessness, and vomiting. On examination, he was conscious, febrile, had tachycardia, and acidotic breathing with a systolic BP of 100 mmHg. His right lower limb was grossly swollen right upto the inguinal ligament and felt like a log of wood. There were erythematous, dusky red patches over the dorsum of the foot and leg. His investigation revealed Hb 9 gm%, TLC 16,800/cu.mm, S creatinine 2.4 mg/dl and plasma glucose of 545 mg% with large amount of ketones in the urine. He denied any history of diabetes mellitus in the past. A clinical diagnosis of freshly detected diabetes, ketoacidosis with infected right lower limb and septicemia was made. He was admitted in the critical care unit and treated with intravenous broad spectrum antibiotics, insulin infusion, and intravenous fluids. After stabilization, he was subjected to fasciotomy with extensive debridement. The surgical decompression extended from the dorsum of the foot to all the compartments of the leg. Swelling over the thigh gradually reduced in 3 days and the patient made a rapid recovery. The wound was regularly cleaned, debrided and dressed at bedside. The wound got covered with red granulation tissue in 4 weeks, after which split skin grafting was carried out (Figs 32.4A to C). On discharge from the hospital, the patient was convinced that his wound healed because of the holy black thread tied around his ankle by his faith healer.

Rapidly progressing necrotizing fascitis is a life threatening situation and can even precipitate ketoacidosis. In the present case, urgent decompression coupled with prompt supportive treatment arrested the disease process and prevented further deterioration. This patient later on could be managed on oral antidiabetics.

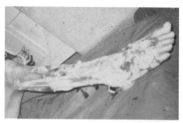

Fig. 32.4A: After extensive fasciotomy extending from dorsum of the leg

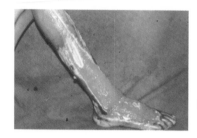

Fig. 32.4B: Granulating wound after 4 weeks

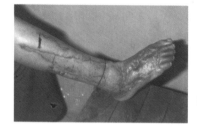

Fig. 32.4C: Wound healed after skin grafting

Case Study (32.B)

This 65 years old female, a housewife, with type 2 DM of 10 years duration, presented with a swollen right upper limb which was accompanied by history of high grade fever since 2 days. There was a history of a small abscess on the dorsum of the right hand. On examination, she was conscious, febrile, had tachycardia, and a systolic BP of 90 mmHg. Her right upper limb was swollen from hand upto the shoulder. There was an abscess on the dorsum of the hand which was draining purulent material with necrosis of the skin over medial aspect of the forearm and arm. Her investigations revealed Hb 9.5 gm%, TLC 18,000/cu.mm, S. creatinine 2.9 gm/dl, ESR 150 mm/1st hour and plasma glucose of 450 mg%. The clinical diagnosis of longstanding DM, necrotizing fascitis of the right upper limb, and septicemia was made.

She was admitted in the critical care unit, switched on to intravenous fluids, broad spectrum antibiotics, and insulin infusion. After stabilizing the clinical condition, she was subjected to surgery. On exploration there was extensive necrosis of the deeper soft tissues both in the forearm and arm. In view of the extensive necrosis, gross infection, and the patient's general condition, the unfortunate decision to carry out shoulder disarticulation was taken and implemented (Fig. 32.5A to 32.5C). The patient had to be given 2 units of blood transfusion intraoperatively, she stood the procedure well and made a rapid recovery.

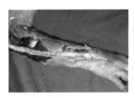

Fig. 32.5A: Fasciotomy right upper limb (dorsal view)

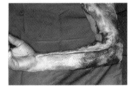

Fig. 32.5B: Fasciotomy right upper limb (medial view)

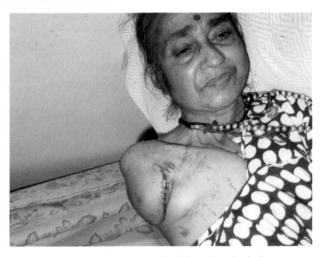

Fig. 32.5C: After right shoulder disarticulation

Case Study (32.C)

This 63 years old male with type 2 DM of 3 years duration and hypothyroidism for which he was on substitution therapy, presented with a swelling and black discoloration of the right foot of 5 days duration following a trivial trauma. On examination, he was febrile, had tachycardia 130/min, BP of 130/76 mmHg. His systemic examination was normal. He had neuropathic feet with normal ABI. Right foot examination revealed patchy, superficial gangrene of the skin involving whole of the dorsum and the 2nd, 3rd and 4th toes. The skin of the great and 5th toes

were apparently normal. On peeling the gangrenous skin, the underlying slough could be seen (Fig. 32.6A). There were similar patches on the plantar aspect. There were also few, small, dusky red areas on the posterior aspect of the skin of the leg. His investigations revealed Hb 11 gm%, TLC 7900/cu.mm, ESR 53 mm/1st hr, S. creatinine 1.8 mg/dl, plasma glucose 365 mg% and HbA$_1$c 10.1%. His duplex Doppler of right lower limb arterial system did not reveal any significant occlusive disease. There was biphasic waveform in the infrapopliteal vessels with dampening of flow in the dorsalis pedis. He was hospitalized, switched on to broad spectrum intravenous antibiotics, multiple injections of insulin and posted for surgery.

Intraoperatively, it was revealed that there was extensive involvement of the deeper tissues and overlying skin of the leg. Because of above reasons, knee disarticulation had to be carried out in place of BK amputation (Fig. 32.6 B).

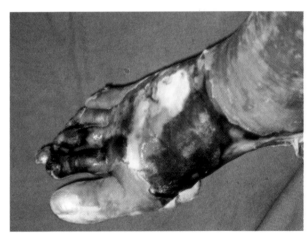

Fig. 32.6A: Right foot showing extensive necrosis within 5 days

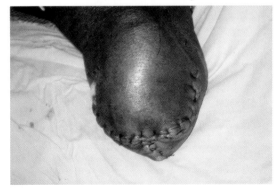

Fig. 32.6B: After right knee disarticulation

33 Life Threatening Infection

One had better lose a limb to earn fresh life

This is the most devastating clinical situation with infected diabetic foot. Deep seated foot infection is no more localized; it has disrupted all the anatomical barriers and has extended proximally, above the ankle, progressing into the leg. The patient with life threatening foot infection, often has a history of foot infection for over one month, has been treated at other places with inadequate, heisitant small incisions, and various antibiotics and has spent few days trying alternative medicine with faith healers. The patient is toxic, debilitated, pale, febrile and has tachycardia. He has extreme weakness, malaise, loss of appetite and vomiting. His laboratory investigations reveal anemia, hypoalbuminemia, chronic hyperglycemia (HbA$_1$c > 9%), hyponatremia, raised total leukocyte counts with erythrocyte sedimentation rates > 100 mm/ 1st hr. Serum creatinine is raised with or without ketonuria. The foot is smelly, bloated and dirty. The foul smell is intolerable and unsuppressible (despite layers of bandages). The foot has a boggy appearance, has multiple openings through which there is a discharge of purulent material and the underlying necrosis is clearly visible. Crepitus (gas in the soft tissue) is often present.

The common reasons for such a galloping foot infection to such an extent, apart from virulent microorganisms and poorly controlled diabetes mellitus, there are medico social factors (Fig. 33.1 to 33.6). These factors are:

* unawareness about diabetic foot and its consequences.
* late reporting
* home surgery
* belief in alternative medicine and faith healers
* continued ambulation despite plantar wound
* small hesitant incisions
* inadequate debridement
* total neglect towards glycemic control
* extra emphasis on expensive antibiotics.

The above mentioned factors are because of ignorance on part of the patient and at times, even the treating doctor. The net result is a culmination into a clinical situation of a life threatening infection. Despite

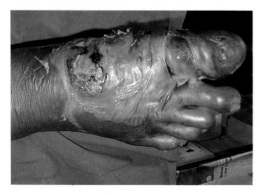

Fig. 33.1: Late reporting, treated with antibiotics, dressings and inadequate debridement resulting in life threatening situation

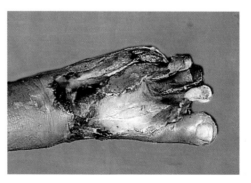

Fig. 33.2: Life threatening situation with extensive necrosis of the foot due to infective process

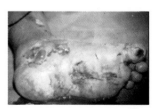

Fig. 33.3: Life threatening foot infection, culprit lesion is in the great toe, note small hesitant incisions, holy thread around the ankle. This patient died soon after this photograph was taken

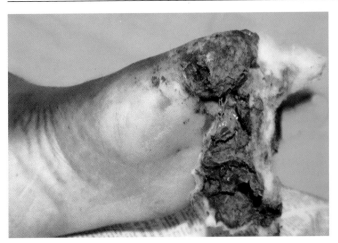

Fig. 33.4: Right great toe packed with herbs, it took a long time to remove it before the great toe could be seen, this patient underwent BK amputation

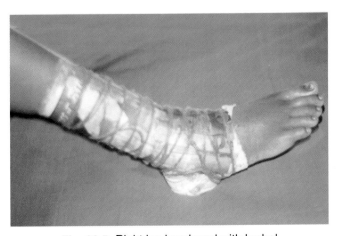

Fig. 33.5: Right leg bandaged with herbal dressing and tied with a coir

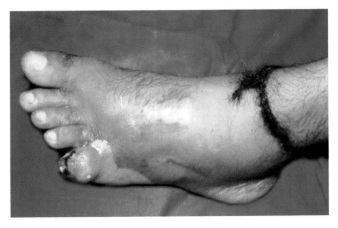

Fig. 33.6: Infected left 5th toe with lateral compartment infection. This patient was treated by a faith healer, who tied a braid made from patient's wife's hair

this critical situation, patient and his family members vehemently refuse the very idea of leg amputation. The patient's refusal for major amputation is a major stumbling block. He moves from one hospital to another in search of a savior who would save his bloated, dirty foot. Such a toxic and moribund patient is a medico-surgical emergency and if the decision of primary leg amputation is not taken promptly, the patient easily progresses to septicemia, shock and multiorgan failure at which stage, even the leg amputation cannot save the patient's life.

MANAGEMENT

The patient with life threatening infection needs to be hospitalized in an intensive care unit. The principles of medical management are similar to those for treatment of limb threatening infection. The patient with life threatening infection needs a major amputation, the site of amputation depends upon the extent of infection and the joint decision of the footcare team. The decision of primary amputation has to be taken and executed at the earliest. Removal of the culprit foot reduces the load of microorganisms and their toxins and patient makes a rapid recovery. Any delay in aggressive medical and surgical treatment, can lead to increased mortality.

It is sad to hear the same old stories from these patients. It also reflects incompetence on part of the medical fraternity for not creating the required awareness among the patients with diabetes mellitus and their treating doctors.

Case Study (33.A)

This 58 years old female with type 2 DM of 9 years duration, presented with history of non-healing wound left foot since 2 months, fever, loss of appetite and weight loss since 4 weeks and hospitalization for last 3 weeks where surgeries on her left foot were carried out. On examination she was toxic, febrile, pale, pulse rate 120/min, BP 100/70 mmHg (Fig. 33.7C). Her systemic examination was however, normal. Examination of feet revealed neuropathy and ABI on right side was normal and the right foot had undergone 5th toe amputation 2 years ago. Her left foot was totally destroyed, stinking and the necrosis had spread into the leg which was edematous, with necrosis of all the visible tendons and muscles (Figs 33.7A and B). Her investigations revealed Hb 5.6 gm%,

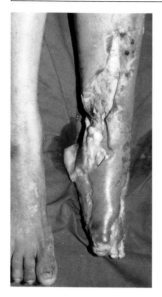

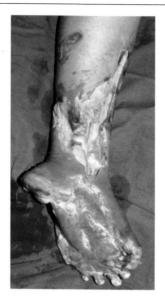

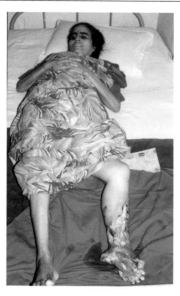

Fig. 33.7A: Life threatening situation left foot and leg,

Fig. 33.7B: Closer view showing extensive destruction of foot and leg

Fig. 33.7C: Pale and pathetic, tense and toxic look of the patient

TLC 16,000/cu.mm, ESR 148 mm/1st hr, S. albumin. 2.5 gms/dl (low) S. Creatinine 2.7 mg/dl, ALT 74 IU/L, AST 68 IU/L, S. Na$^+$ 126 mEq/L, S. K$^+$ 4.1 mEq/L, plasma glucose 448 mg% and HbA$_1$c of 10.8%.

A clinical diagnosis of type 2 DM, advanced left foot and leg infection, severe anemia, hypoproteinemia, toxic hepatitis, prerenal insufficiency, septicemia was made. She was advised AK amputation, after stabilization of clinical condition. The patient and her close relations were totally against amputation and wanted us to salvage the limb. Despite explaining that the limb was beyond salvage and above knee amputation would be life saving, they took her to another hospital. Three weeks later, she underwent AK amputation but died the very next day of multiorgan failure.

Salvaging the foot is not always possible and has its own limitations. The anatomical extent of the infection, vascular status of the limb, general condition of the patient and results of biochemical and other investigations are the factors which help to reach a decision of salvage or amputation. Timely amputation can prove to be life saving. In this patient, AK amputation could have saved her life, had it been done a few weeks earlier.

Case Study (33.B)

This 44 years old male with type 2 DM of 6 years duration and hypertension since 4 years, presented with longstanding non-healing wound over right foot, since 3 months, fever since 1 month, nausea and weight loss. Three months ago, he had sustained an injury to the right foot after which it was swollen and red. He had received antibiotics. Two weeks later there was discoloration of the great toe and foul smelling discharge. He was operated elsewhere, where debridement over the dorsum of the foot was performed with a small incision over the medial plantar aspect. Despite surgery, patient's general condition continued to deteriorate, so also the wound. At this stage, he was referred to our centre.

On examination, his general condition was not satisfactory, he was pale, febrile, pulse rate 130/min, BP 130/70 mmHg. His systemic examination was normal. He had neuropathic feet and ABI was normal on left but could not be assessed on the right because of swelling. The right foot showed gangrene of the great toe, diffuse swelling of the plantar aspect especially medial aspect with a small scar of previous debridement through which necrotic tissue was visible and it discharged purulent material on pressure (Fig. 33.8B). Dorsally there was evidence of debridement through which necrotic muscles and tendons were seen (Fig. 33.8A). The whole foot was erythematous and swollen and discharged pus on pressure. The leg was swollen right up to knee joint and there were dusky red patches on the leg skin. The right femoral artery was palpable without any bruit on auscultation.

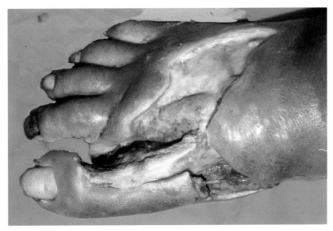

Fig. 33.8A: Dorsal view right foot showing extensive destruction with marks of previous debridement

tachycardia. X-ray of the foot showed destruction of the phalanges of the great toe and 1st MTP joint. Duplex Doppler of right lower limb arterial system did not show any occlusive disease except for dampening of blood flow in the foot because of cellulitis. He was switched on to intravenous broad spectrum antibiotics, intravenous fluid therapy, insulin infusion, blood transfusion and was posted for surgery. In view of longstanding wound, compromised clinical condition and extensive destruction of foot with evidence of spread into the leg, a decision to carry out AK amputation was taken and implemented (Fig. 33.8C).

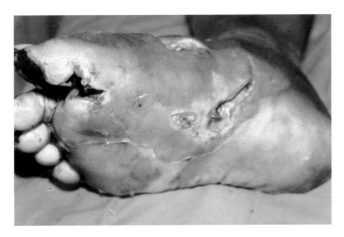

Fig. 33.8B: Plantar view showing necrosis and destruction of the foot with evidence of inadequate debridement

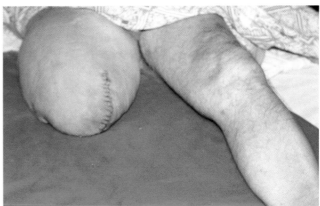

Fig. 33.8C: The patient required AK amputation

A clinical diagnosis of type 2 DM, hypertension, advanced foot infection extending into the leg, anemia and septicemia was made. He was admitted in critical care unit and investigated. His Hb 7.4 gm%, TLC 19,400/cu.mm, hematocrit 24%, ESR 149 mm/1st hr, S. Creatinine 2.4 mg/dl, ALT 150 IU/L, AST 61 IU/L, S. Albumin 2.3 gm/dl, S. Na$^+$ 126 mEq/L, S. K$^+$ 4.1 mEq/L, plasma glucose 470 mg% and HbA$_1$c 10.6%, urine albumin was (++++). His ECG showed sinus

The patient made gradual recovery, fever subsided, appetite improved and he was weaned off intravenous fluids. Rehabilitation was started 5 days after the surgery. One month later his Hb was 10.5 gm%, hematocrit 39%, TLC 10,400/cu.mm, ESR 64 mm/1st hr and S. creatinine 0.6 mg/dl. He was discharged after 6 weeks of hospitalization.

Four years later, he went into chronic renal failure and eventually died of metabolic complications.

Neuroischemic Foot

- Clinical Signs and Symptoms of Ischemia

- Medial Arterial Calcification (Monckeberg's Sclerosis)

- Evaluation of Neuroischemic Foot

- Management of Neuroischemic Foot

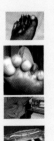

34 Clinical Signs and Symptoms of Ischemia

Cold and Bald, Painful and Pulseless

Although atherosclerosis in patients with diabetes is similar to that seen in nondiabetics, it is generalized, occurs prematurely and progresses at an accelerated pace. Coronary artery, cerebrovascular and peripheral vascular disease (PVD) are the predominant manifestations of macrovascular disease in diabetes. Majority of patients with PVD have associated coronary artery disease, however the opposite is not true. This is perhaps because the clinical manifestations of PVD occur almost a decade later than those of coronary artery disease. In fact the disease of posterior tibial artery commonly seen in diabetics, is a surrogate marker of coronary artery disease.

Peripheral vascular disease in diabetics differs from that in non diabetics, in many ways as shown in Table 34.1.

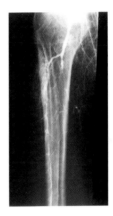

Fig. 34.1: Conventional angiography showing diffuse occlusive disease in the femoral vessels of a diabetic

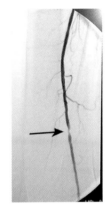

Fig. 34.2: DSA showing isolated block in the lower part of superficial femoral artery of a nondiabetic

Table 34.1: Differences in PVD between diabetics and nondiabetics (Fig. 34.1, 34.2).

Characteristics	Diabetic	Nondiabetic
Clinical	Common	Less common
	Young age	Older age
	Course more rapid	Course less rapid
Male/Female	M > F	M >>> F
Occlusion	Multisegmental	Single segment
Vessels adjacent to occlusion	Involved	Not involved
Collateral vessels	Involved	Usually normal
Lower extremities	Usually bilateral	Unilateral
Vessels involved	Proximal and distal	Proximal

PREVALENCE

The prevalence of PVD is low in Asians as compared to Caucasians (4% vs 20%), probably because of the younger age and shorter duration of diabetes among Asians. The prevalence increases with age and duration of diabetes, it is 3.2% in those below 50 years of age and increases to 33% in those above 80 years.

Similarly, it is 15% at 10 years after the initial diagnosis of type 2 diabetes and jumps to 45% at 20 years duration of diabetes.

Risk factors for development of PVD are the same as those for macrovascular disease in diabetics like genetic predisposition, age, duration of hyperglycemia, smoking, hypertension, dyslipidemia, central obesity, insulin resistance, proteinuria and dialysis.

Peripheral vascular disease is found at all levels of the arterial tree (Fig. 34.3), but atheroma has an apparent predilection for certain sites, namely at bifurcation

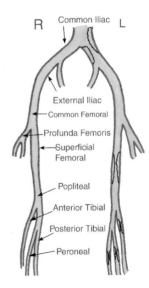

Fig. 34.3: Arterial tree of lower limb vessels showing areas commonly occluded in diabetics

and bends in the artery where hemodynamic shear stress is low or flow separation occurs. In lower limb the common sites are the aortoiliac segment and superficial femoral artery (SFA) in the adductor canal. In diabetics more distal vessels like, tibials and peroneals are commonly involved.

CLINICAL SYMPTOMS

Peripheral vascular disease in diabetics is relatively oligosymptomatic as compared to nondiabetics and hence the diagnosis is often delayed. Often a history of claudication in diabetic patients leads directly to the unheralded appearance of nonhealing wounds or gangrene. The associated neuropathy in diabetics, often masks some of the symptoms of PVD, similar to silent myocardial infarction, thus misleading the treating physician. The classification of PVD based mainly on symptoms is depicted below.

Fontaine Classification

Stage 1 : Occlusive arterial disease without symptoms.
Stage 2 : Intermittent claudication
Stage 3 : Ischemic rest pain
Stage 4 : Ulceration / gangrene

Claudication is the most important symptom of PVD. The presenting symptoms are weakness, cramps, pain or fatigue of exercised muscles while walking and prompt relief on rest. Although very specific in its presentation, occasionally it can be difficult to differentiate from the 'pseudoclaudication syndrome' of lumbar canal stenosis. The characteristics of vascular disease are prompt relief on rest and the reproducibility of the symptoms on walking, while patients with pseudoclaudication must sit or lie down to obtain relief.

The presence of critical narrowing in the peripheral artery is related to the severity of stenosis (fixed) and volume of crossing blood flow (variable). Claudication occurs when muscular activity increases the demand of blood flow by upto 20 folds over resting state, as the vessel with critical stenosis fails to meet the increased demand. Cessation of exercise leads to restoration of situation and disappearance of the pain.

The level of vascular obstruction can be judged by the muscle groups producing the symptoms of claudication. Claudication in the buttocks indicates a block in the terminal aorta, thigh claudication a disease of the iliac arteries, calf claudication suggests disease of the femorals and fatigue and pain in foot indicates obstructive disease of the calf vessels (tibials and peroneal).

Worsening of the vascular disease can be judged by the shortening in distance of claudication, from walking three blocks to walking only one block, eventually leading to rest pain (critical leg ischemia). Rest pain is the prominent complaint in limb threatening ischemia and usually signifies advanced vascular disease with critical stenosis. It is more on lying supine because it eliminates the gravity, contributing to perfusion and a slight drop in blood pressure during sleep further aggravates it. Ischemic pain arouses the patient from sleep who gets relief by walking a few steps. This probably elevates the blood pressure, restores the gravity effect, thus improving the perfusion. Frequently patients with severe rest pain sleep in chairs with their feet in dependent position to eliminate discomfort. Worsening of vascular disease can lead to painful ulcerations on foot or black discoloration of toes or part of foot.

Acute onset ischemic pain can occur as a result of embolism. Immediate referral to an interventional radiologist and vascular surgeon is warranted for institution of intraarterial thrombolytic therapy and or emergency vascular surgery like embolectomy.

CLINICAL SIGNS

Evaluation of the lower extremity and examination of foot are extremely important. The fundamental of examination, i.e. palpation of peripheral pulses is often not done. The palpation of femoral, popliteal, posterior tibial and dorsalis pedis pulses should be carried out and graded as normal, diminished or absent. Auscultation of femoral and aortoiliac regions for a bruit, should be performed. Bruit occurs at areas of arterial narrowing, with onset around 50% stenosis and disappearance around 90% stenosis. Examination of the foot can reveal diminished temperature and hair growth, dependent rubor, discoloration of toes, dystrophic nails (Fig. 34.4), or tender ulceration on the margins of toes. Dependent rubor results from vasodilatation secondary to ischemia (Fig. 34.5) and indicates significant vascular disease.

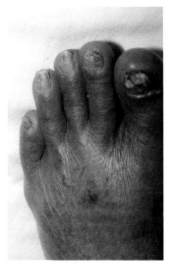

Fig. 34.4: Ischemic foot, note dystrophic nails, loss of hair

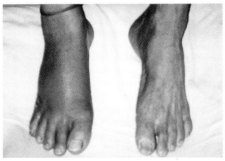

Fig. 34.5: Dependent rubor right foot

Capillary Refill Time

In supine position, pressure is applied to the skin and once removed the reappearance of normal skin color occurs within 5 seconds, it gets delayed in vascular disease.

Venous Refill Time

Can be determined by identifying prominent veins on the dorsum of foot. In supine position, the leg is then elevated 45 degrees for one minute, following which the patient sits up and hangs the leg over the side of the examination table. The time in seconds between assuming the upright position and reappearance of the vein bulging above the skin level is recorded. The normal venous refill time is 20 seconds or less.

Chronic Critical Leg Ischemia

It is currently defined as persistent rest pain requiring regular analgesia for more than two weeks and/or ulceration or gangrene of the foot or toes, both associated with an ankle systolic pressure of < 50 mmHg. or toe systolic pressure of < 30 mmHg.

Gangrene

Gangrene is the endpoint of PVD and denotes necrosis of the skin and underlying tissues, thus indicating an irreversible damage where healing cannot be anticipated without loss of some part of the extremity. Gangrene can be wet or dry.

Wet Gangrene

The tissues are grey or black, moist and often malodorus, affected part is swollen and the epidermis may be raised in blebs, adjoining tissues are infected and pus may discharge from ulcerated areas. Wet gangrene denotes severe soft tissue infection with advanced PVD (Fig. 34.6, 34.7). Association of infection and ischemic foot is a deadly combination and carries a bad prognosis.

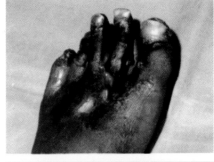

Fig. 34.6: Wet gangrene left foot, note swelling and ulceration

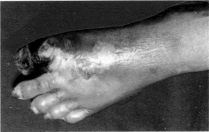

Fig. 34.7: Left foot great toe gangrene with infection

Dry Gangrene

The tissues are hard, blackened, mummified and there is usually a clean line of demarcation between the necrotic and viable tissues (Fig. 34.8). Dry gangrene results from severe ischemia secondary to poor tissue perfusion, from atherosclerotic narrowing of the arteries of the leg, complicated by thrombosis and embolization. Its presentation is usually chronic but rarely can be of an acute onset. It is free from infection.

Early diagnosis of PVD is extremely important, as institution of medical therapy and reduction of the risk factors can go a long way in preventing much of the morbidity and even the mortality.

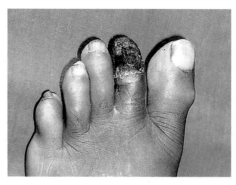

Fig. 34.8: Dry gangrene left foot 2nd toe, note the line of demarcation

35 Medial Arterial Calcification (Monckeberg's Sclerosis)

Vessels are like a "Lead-pipe"

Monckeberg's sclerosis or medial arterial calcification is degenerative arteriosclerosis of the peripheral arteries characterized by fibrotic and calcific changes involving intimal plaque and media. Intermediate sized muscular arteries are commonly involved. The vessels are in compressible (lead pipe) and thus elevate ankle systolic blood pressure. The ankle/brachial systolic blood pressure index is falsely elevated above 1.2.

Medial calcification is seen in about 20 to 25% of patients with longstanding type two diabetes. It is commonly associated with autonomic neuropathy and renal insufficiency. Calcification of the vessels does not signify occlusive vascular disease although, both can be associated. The atherosclerotic lesions are found in the intimal layer of the arterial wall while calcification occurs near the internal elastic membrane with little or no effect on the lumen of the vessel.

Clinical suspicion of medial calcification of vessels is made when ABI is found to be above 1.2. The diagnosis can be confirmed on plain radiography. Radiographically, intimal calcifications are distributed in an irregular fashion along the vessel wall (tram lines). It can be seen in abdominal aorta, femoral and tibial vessels on plain radiography (Fig. 35.1 to 35.4). It can also been seen in foot vessels, although less frequently than tibial vessels. Medial calcification is

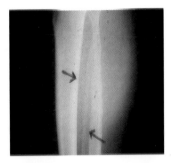

Fig. 35.2: Calcification in leg artery

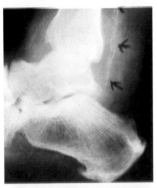

Fig. 35.3: Calcification in the tibial artery

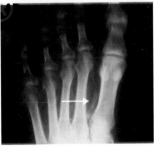

Fig. 35.4: Calcification in a foot vessel

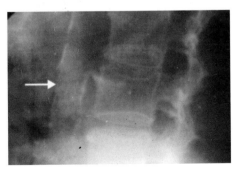

Fig. 35.1: Calcification in the abdominal aorta

common in proximal than distal vessels with a clear gradient from proximal to distal, which is in contrast to the distal-to-proximal gradient of peripheral neuropathy.

Case Study (35.A)

This 72 year old male a nonsmoker, with type 2 DM of 10 years, presented with non healing wound left foot, since 15 days. On inspection it looked to be an advanced neuroischemic foot with necrotic skin over the dorsum and gangrene of the 4th toe (35.5 A, 35.5 D). The dorsalis pedis artery wasn't located, however posterior tibial artery was felt. While recording his ABI, the posterior tibial artery could not be obliterated even upto 300 mmHg., whereas his brachial systolic pressure was 140 mmHg. Thus the ABI was > 2 suggestive of Monckeberg's sclerosis. His X-ray of the

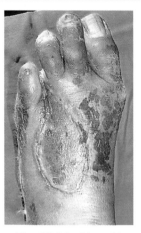

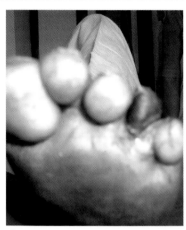

Fig. 35.5C: After skin grafting

Fig. 35.5D: Plantar aspect shows gangrene of 4th toe and swelling

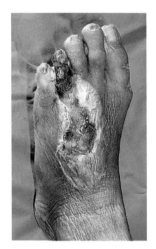

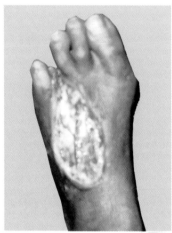

Fig. 35.5A: At presentation note gangrene of 4th toe and necrosis of skin over dorsum

Fig. 35.5B: After radical debridement and disarticulation of 4th toe

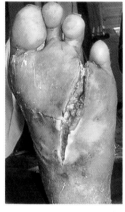

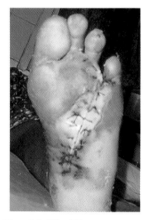

Fig. 35.5E: Deep plantar incision to remove necrotic tissue

Fig. 35.5F: Plantar wound closed by secondary suturing

leg revealed arterial calcification. Duplex Doppler revealed thickening of the arterial walls with loss of triphasic waveform in the popliteal and infrapopliteal vessels without any stenotic lesions. Vascular surgeon was consulted, who ruled out any surgical intervention. The patient was taken for surgical debridement of the wound. The dorsal gangrenous skin was excised, 4th toe disarticulated at MTP joint and through an extended and deep plantar incision, necrotic and infected material was removed (Fig. 35.5 B, 35.5 E). Three weeks later, the patient underwent split skin grafting for the dorsal wound and secondary suturing of the plantar defect (Fig. 35.5 C, 35.5 F).

Although, it looked like a case of advanced PVD, it was more of infective arteritis causing digital necrosis. Monckeberg's sclerosis was an incidental finding.

36 Evaluation of Neuroischemic Foot

Pray the amputation guillotine falls less often

There are several invasive and noninvasive methods to evaluate the neuroischemic foot. The critical assessment areas are; prediction of wound healing, decide on the need for revascularization and/or to judge the correct level for amputation.

ANKLE/BRACHIAL PRESSURE INDEX (ABI)

A hand-held Doppler can be used to confirm the presence of pulses and to quantify the vascular supply. When used together with sphygmomanometer, the ankle and brachial systolic pressures are measured and their ratio calculated (Fig. 36.1) . In normal subjects, the ankle systolic pressure is higher than the brachial systolic pressure. Normal ABI is > 1 and in presence of ischemia it is < 0.9. Absent or feeble peripheral pulses with ABI <0.9 confirms ischemia. Conversly, the presence of pulses and ABI of > 1 rules out significant ischemia. In medial arterial calcification (Monckeberg's Sclerosis), the calcified arteries being incompressible, the ABI is falsely elevated > 1.2. An ABI of <0.5 indicates significant ischemia and further evaluation like angiography is warranted.

TOE SYSTOLIC PRESSURE (TSP)

Toe pressures can be measured using special pressure cuffs and have been found useful in predicting the clinical course of rest pain or skin ulcerations. TSP of less than 40 mm Hg signifies significant ischemia.

TRANSCUTANEOUS PRESSURE OF OXYGEN TENSION (TcPO₂)

$TcPO_2$ is a noninvasive method for monitoring arterial oxygen tension and reflects local arterial perfusion pressure (Fig. 36.2). A heated oxygen sensitive probe is placed on the dorsum of the foot and a reference probe below the clavicle. After an equilibrium period of 15 minutes, the skin oxygen tension (mm Hg) is determined, which reflects local blood flow. Normal values are usualy > 60 mmHg, a level below 30 mm Hg. indicates severe ischemia but levels can be falsely lowered by edema or cellulitis.

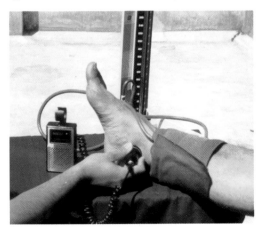

Fig. 36.1: Ankle pressure measurement by a hand-held Doppler

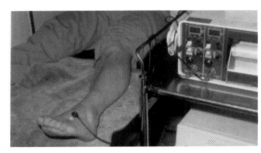

Fig. 36.2: Measurement of $TcPO_2$ (*Courtesy*, ME Edmonds, AVM Foster, King's College Hospital, London, UK)

Ankle systolic pressure (P ankle), TSP, and $TcPO_2$ help predict the probability of the wound healing (see Table 36.1)

Table 36.1: Probability of foot ulcer healing			
Test	Absolute pressure (mmHg)	Diabetic patients (%)	Non-diabetic patients (%)
1. P ankle	≤ 55	Unlikely	Unlikely
	55-90	45	85
	≥ 90	85	100
2. P toe	≤ 30	45	70
	30-50	75	100
	≥ 55	95	100
3. TcPo2	≥ 40	Likely	Likely
TcPo2	≤ 20	unlikely	unlikely

P ankle, ankle pressure; P toe, toe pressure; TcPO$_2$, transcutaneous pressure of oxygen (Ref. No. 7)

DUPLEX COLOUR DOPPLER

It is an invaluable tool in the diagnostic evaluation of the peripheral vascular tree. Normal lower limb arteries, on Doppler, show a triphasic wave pattern (Fig. 36.3). This consists of a strong peak systolic notch, followed by a slight reversal of flow during early diastole and return to forward flow of low amplitude or diastolic run off. In atherosclerotic occlusive disease, this normal triphasic pattern is changed. There

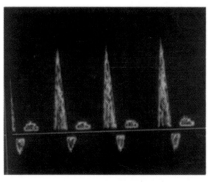

Fig. 36.3: Normal triphasic wave form

is an increased peak systolic velocity, and absent early diastolic reversal producing a biphasic wave form (Fig. 36.4). Further stenosis causes disappearance of the diastolic run-off, giving monophasic wave form (Fig. 36.5). In the presence of significant stenosis, there is a

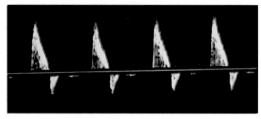

Fig. 36.4: Biphasic wave form

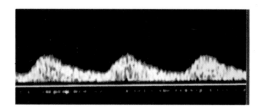

Fig. 36.5: Monophasic wave form with dampened flow

high peak systolic velocity proximal to and a dampened peak systolic velocity distal to the stenosis. Good collaterals development results in resumption of the diastolic flow distal to the stenosis, while acute thromboembolism shows absence of flow. Calcification in the vessel wall is seen in the form of flow turbulence and high reflectivity index. Duplex Doppler can detect hemodynamically significant stenosis and extent of the atherosclerotic vascular disease in the major lower limb vessels upto the begining of the plantar arch.

Duplex Doppler is useful whenever bypass graft surgery is contemplated. Prior to surgery, it is useful to identify a suitable vein, its size, patency and evidence of varicosities. The course of the vein (great saphenous) can be mapped on the skin. Duplex Doppler is also useful to identify run off arteries suitable for use in vascular reconstruction. After surgery it helps to identify stenosis, thrombosis, mismatches in lumen size and abnormal flow patterns in the bypass graft. Regular monitoring permits early intervention to prolong graft life and to enhance limb salvage rate.

The advantages of duplex Doppler are, it is non invasive, less expensive and can be repeated several times. Despite all the advantages, it is certainly not a substitute for angiography. The limitations of duplex Doppler are difficulty in assessing obese individuals, under-evaluation of multiple narrowings, under-estimation of the degree of narrowings and difficulty in detecting early vessel wall narrowing.

INTRAVASCULAR ULTRASOUND (IVUS)

The attachment of ultrasound transducers to catheters has created a completely new modality, intravascular ultrasound (IVUS), which can evaluate vessels "from inside out". IVUS determines percentage of stenosis, confirms dissection and evaluates vessel walls and plaques. It has a potential to play an adjunctive role in complex endovascular interventions involving angioplasty and stents.

COMPUTERIZED TOMOGRAPHY ANGIOGRAPHY (CTA)

Spiral CT is rapidly replacing conventional CT imaging. One advantage, besides the speed of scanning, is its ability to generate three-dimensional (3-D) images. CT angioraphy (CTA) (Fig. 36.6, 36.7) is an important application of the 3-D capabilities of spiral CT. CTA is more useful in large arteries such as thoracic or abdominal aorta but its disadvantages are need of intravascular administration of contrast and the inability to accurately assess smaller vessels. In diabetics, commonly involved vessels are infrapopliteal, which are not properly assessed by CTA, thus limiting its immediate application.

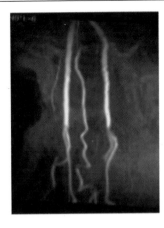

Fig. 36.8: MR angiography showing block in profunda femoris left

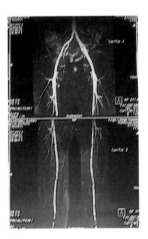

Fig. 36.6: 3D reconstruction of CT angiography showing vascular tree of lower limbs

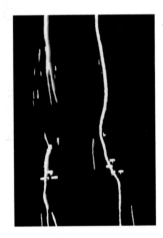

Fig. 36.7: CT angiography showing a long segment block in superficial femoral left, with reformation of popliteal through collaterals

MAGNETIC RESONANCE ANGIOGRAPHY (MRA)

MRA is arguably the most dwarfing imaging development in the recent past and not just in the evaluation of extra and intracranial carotid circulation. The advantages of MRA are, the procedure is simple, quick and non renal toxic. It has a potential to accurately assess peripheral vessels and distal pedal arteries for surgical bypass in diabetics (Fig. 36.8). In the light of rapid advances in technology, MRA is well poised to soon replace contrast angiography as a primary screening procedure with the latter then

reserved for more demanding and finer diagnostic and therapeutic procedures.

ANGIOGRAPHY

Transfemoral angiography is the gold standard for evaluation of PVD in diabetics (Fig. 36.9). Due to increased incidence of nephrotoxicity in the diabetic population, minimal radiographic contrast administration, combined with adequate hydration prior to and after the procedure, is mandatory. It is also advisable to avoid metformin (oral hypoglycemic agent) 48 hours prior to and subsequent to the use of parentral contrast agents, to avoid the risk of lactic acidosis and nephrotoxicity. Another strategy to reduce contrast load is to perform isolated angiography of the symptomatic limb if the unaffected limb has been found to be normal on physical examination and non invasive tests.

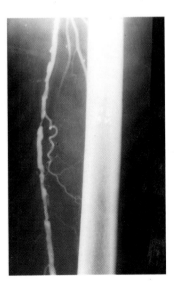

Fig. 36.9: Conventional angiogram showing diffuse narrowing in superficial femoral artery left

Digital Subtraction Angiography (DSA)

DSA is now the state of art and has largely replaced conventional angiography. It is able to produce excellent angiograms even in the distal pedal circulation with a minimal amount of contrast (Fig. 36.10). DSA is helpful in calculating the diameter of the inflow vessel and degree as well as length of stenosis.

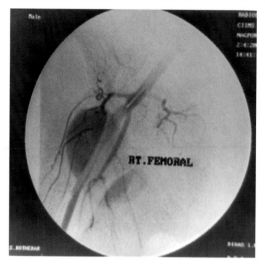

Fig. 36.11: DSA showing pseudoaneurysm near right femoral artery, a post angiography complication

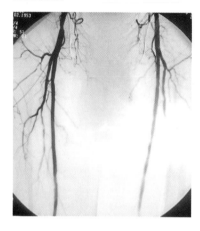

Fig. 36.10: DSA showing narrowing in left superficial femoral, note DSA picture is after subtraction of soft tissue and bones

The advantages of DSA are:
- Less contrast is required
- Superior contrast resolution
- Shorter procedure time
- Data can be stored and processed later
- Images show only the arteries, not bones and soft tissues.

Despite the high degree of sensitivity, DSA angiography may fail to opacify distal peripheral arteries, especially when advanced PVD is present. This could be disadvantageous for the vascular surgeon who is contemplating a distal vascular bypass. Although angiography (conventional and DSA) are relatively safe procedures, they do carry a significant morbidity especially in patients with old age, longstanding diabetes, renal impairment and severe vascular disease.

Potential complications of angiography are :
- Puncture site thrombosis
- Pseudoaneurysm (Fig. 36.11)
- Dissection
- Arteriovenous fistula
- Distal embolization
- Spasm of the vessel
- Nephrotoxicity
- Allergic reaction

Most diabetics with PVD have a significant occlusive disease in the popliteal artery or below the trifurcation (tibials and peroneal). The evaluation of neuroischemic foot should give information about level of the stenotic lesion, degree of stenosis, length of the occluded vessel and status of vessels proximal and distal to occlusion. The vascular surgeon is also interested in knowing the proximal inflow of the vessel and distal reformation of the vessels. On the basis of this information, he can plan either an angioplasty or bypass surgery to salvage the limb, or decide the level of leg amputation.

37 Management of Neuroischemic Foot

Prior to a major amputation, always consult a vascular surgeon

The clinical course of peripheral vascular disease in diabetics is associated with a premature onset, rapid progression and often involvement of both the limbs. It is therefore prudent to evaluate every patient suspected to have vascular insufficiency and to take appropriate steps to aggressively treat the associated risk factors, offer medical treatment or vascular reconstruction as per the merits of the case. Once ulceration or gangrene occurs, the prognosis worsens rapidly; such patients often require limb amputation or even a contralateral limb amputation in a couple of years with its associated morbidity and mortality.

NONPHARMACOLOGICAL THERAPY

The two most important modalities are walking as an exercise and abstinence from smoking. These measures increase the claudication distance thus promoting pain free ambulation. The value of footcare should be emphasized, with a special reference to treatment of interdigital mycosis, prevention of dryness, and cracking of the feet, wearing comfortable shoes, maintaining good foot hygiene and a proper nail care. Associated risk factors like dyslipidemia and hypertension should be promptly treated. The use of b blockers should be avoided.

PHARMACOLOGICAL THERAPY

A variety of drugs are being used, to treat peripheral vascular disease, like vasodilators, statins, antiplatelet, anticoagulants, hemorrheologic, and thrombolytic agents; the rationale being to increase oxygen delivery or improve utilization of oxygen in ischemic tissues. Patients with PVD are already maximally vasodilated (auto-sympathectomy) reducing the need for vasodilators. However, there is some evidence of clinical benefits with the use of calcium channel blocker, Verapamil. Antiplatelet agents including aspirin, ticlopidine, dipyridamole, clopidogrel and prostacyclin (PGI_2) have been extensively studied, because of the key role played by platelets in arterial thrombosis and atherosclerosis. Although there has not been any significant symptomatic improvement with their use, they are usually administered because they slow the progression of atherosclerotic disease. Statins are given for their lipid lowering effect and other actions like, a decrease in the thrombus formation, improvement in endothelial function, and inhibition of platelet aggregation.

We have seen improvement in the ambulatory walking distance and even a reversal from monophasic to the normal triphasic waveform in duplex Doppler with daily injections of low molecular weight heparin for 3 to 4 weeks in Fontaine's class 2 and 3 patients. Pentoxifylline, a hemorrheologic drug has been also tried and has been found to be moderately effective in increasing the claudication distance and giving some relief in the ischemic rest pain. It must be remembered that pharmacological therapy has a limited role to play in an established case of neuro-ischemic foot.

LUMBAR SYMPATHECTOMY

In patients with diabetes, there is already an autosympathectomy as a result of associated autonomic neuropathy. Therefore lumbar sympathectomy is not really warranted.

THROMBOLYTIC THERAPY

It is of special importance in an acute onset ischemia. Local infiltration of a thrombolytic agent into the thrombus using a catheter, requires lower doses and is therefore, probably safer than systemic therapy. Urokinase gives better results than streptokinase. Thrombolysis functions best in an acute thrombosis including acutely occluded grafts. A balloon dilatation is often necessary after the thrombolysis, to dilate an underlying stenosis. Some workers prefer to use thrombolytic therapy before balloon dilatation for old occlusions as they often contain some lysable material. Prostanoids, prostaglandin I_2 (PGI_2), E_1 (PGE_1), prostacycline analogue, and platelet receptor antagonist (GpIIb/IIa)have also been tried, in the treatment of acute thrombosis, with beneficial results. A newer technique to instill thrombolytic agent is pulse spray technique, which by its virtue of spray also causes mechanical thrombolysis.

PERCUTANEOUS TRANSLUMINAL ANGIOPLASTY (PTA)

The last two decades have witnessed an explosion in radiographically monitored percutaneous catheter techniques, referred to as endovascular procedures to treat vascular stenosis or in some cases, even occlusions. The most common of these catheter-based procedures is balloon dilatation angioplasty (Fig. 37.1). In addition to balloon angioplasty, a variety of other endovascular procedures are available including laser angioplasty, mechanical atherectomy, and intra-vascular stents. These procedures have advantages in that there is a reduced hospital stay, a reduction in the frequency of complications, low mortality, high success, and patency rate. However, to date the follow up has been short and as such the long-term durability of endovascular procedures for PVD are unknown.

Success of angioplasty depends upon the morphology and character of the stenotic lesions. Ideal lesions for angioplasty are short (≤ 10 cm), concentric, non-ostial, and non-calcified. Patients with suboptimal results after a balloon angioplasty can now be treated with endovascular stents. In PVD, angioplasty can be carried out with optimal results in aortoiliac (Fig. 37.2 A to 37.2 C), femoral (Fig. 37.3 A, 37.3 B), and poplitial

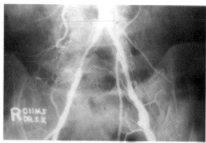

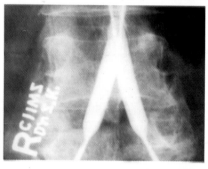

Fig. 37.2A: Stenotic lesions both common iliac arteries

Fig. 37.2B: Kissing angioplasty

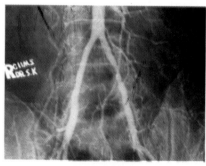

Fig. 37.2C: Stenotic lesions reopened ofter angioplasty

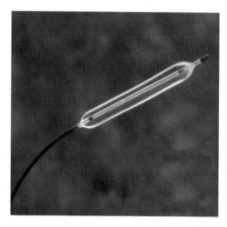

Fig. 37.1: Balloon dilatation catheter

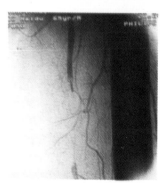

Fig. 37.3A: DSA showing complete block in superficial femoral artery

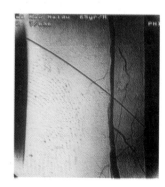

Fig. 37.3B: After balloon dilatation angioplasty, the vessel has been reopened

arteries (Fig. 37.4 A to 37.4 C), and with the availability of smaller balloon catheters, even smaller stenotic vessels below the trifurcation such as the tibials and peroneal (characteristic of a diabetic PVD), can be opened up (Fig. 37.5A to 37.5D). Percutaneous transluminal angioplasty and stents have been an excellent addition in the management of PVD in diabetics. These endovascular procedures are also indicated in solitary lesions, after a thrombolytic therapy in an acute ischemia, and as a complimentary procedure to limb salvage surgery or vascular bypass surgery. However, dissection, thrombosis, spasm and vessel recoil can be some of the complications of angioplasty.

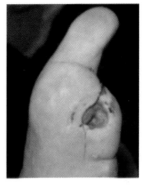
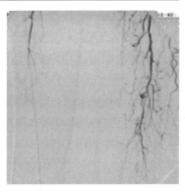

Fig. 37.5A: *69 years old male with a history of resection of the second through fourth toe with subplantar abscess underwent angiography

Fig. 37.5B: *Angiography showed short segment occlusion of the superficial femoral artery and multiple crural occlusions

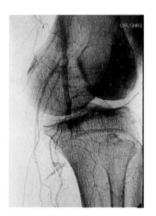
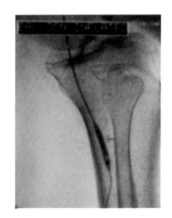

Fig. 37.4A: Angiography showing complete occlusion in the popliteal artery

Fig. 37.4B: Balloon dilatation catheter in position

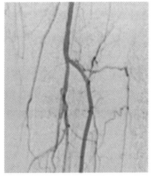
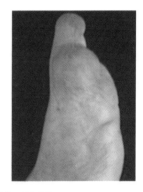

Fig. 37.5C: *Percutaneous transluminal angioplasty (PTA) of the distal superficial femoral artery was performed

Fig. 37.5D: *Wound healing after sucessful PTA

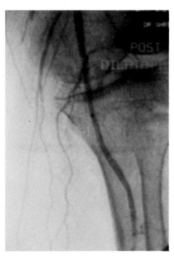

Fig. 37.4C: *Popliteal artery reopened after angioplasty*

A rapidly advancing technology is certainly going to see angioplasty and stenting as the procedures of first choice for vascular lesion in coronaries, cerebral, renal and even peripheral vessels. However, diabetics do not seem to be ideal candidates for peripheral angioplasty and stenting procedures, because of generalized, diffuse, and often bilateral involvement with specific affliction of infra-popliteal vessels.

THE ROLE OF VASCULAR SURGERY

Diabetics are unique in their propensity to develop severe infra-inguinal disease with relative sparing of the aorto-iliac vessels. The most severely affected vessels are often the sub-trifurcation crural arteries, the anterior tibial, posterior tibial, and peroneal vessels with sparing of the arteries of the foot (Figs 37.6, 37.7).

* Reproduced by kind permission by the International Working Group on the Diabetic Foot

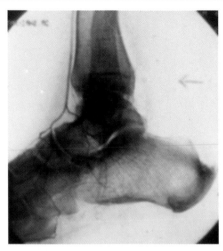

Fig. 37.6: Angiography showing complete block in posterior tibial artery, anterior tibial normal

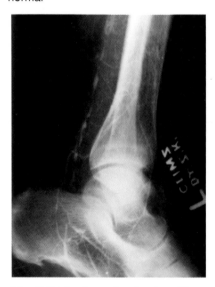

Fig. 37.7: Angiography showing diffuse occlusive disease in posterior tibial artery, reformation of plantar vessels through anterior tibial artery

This pattern of occlusive disease requires a different approach to vascular reconstruction and presents special challenges for the vascular surgeon. As the vascular bypass surgery in lower limbs in associated with significant morbidity and even mortality, it is essential to screen these patients before any surgery is planned.

Indications for Vascular Surgery in Lower Limb

- Severely disabling intermittent claudication
- Critical leg ischemia (Limb threatening)
- Nonhealing ischemic foot ulcers or distal gangrene.

Contraindications for Vascular Surgery

- Chronically bedridden patients
- The very old
- Those with organic brain syndrome
- Flexion contractures of the knee
- Patients with significant multisystem diseases.

As PVD in diabetics is invariably associated with coronary artery disease, although the reverse is not true, a proper evaluation of the cardiac status is extremely important before lower limb bypass surgery. The vascular surgery should be delayed in patients with an ischemic ulcer and secondary foot infection, until the clinical signs of infection like fever, cellulitis, and lymphangitis have improved.

Principles of Vascular Surgery

The ultimate goal of lower extremity arterial reconstruction is to restore perfusion pressure in the distal circulation, by bypassing all major occlusions and if possible, reestablishing a palpable foot pulse. The recipient artery (distal to the block), usually dorsalis pedis, anterior tibial, or posterior tibial and the donor artery (proximal to the block), usually the femoral or popliteal vessel, should be relatively free of an occlusive disease. The conduit used is the saphenous vein. It can be harvested for use as a reversed saphenous vein graft, wherein the distal end of the vein (smaller diameter) is anastomosed to the larger donor artery (femoral). The risk of thrombosis of the vein graft in these cases is more because of size discrepancy. A newer technique is to use the saphenous vein "in situ" by dividing the venous valves (Fig. 37.8) to permit a proximal to distal flow, and ligating the venous tributaries to prevent arterio-

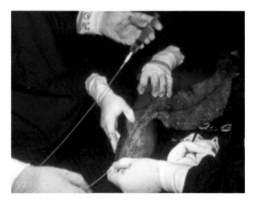

Fig. 37.8: Valvulotome being used to divide the venous valves

venous fistulae. The proximal and distal ends of the vein are then anastomosed with a better size match, to the donor and recipient arteries, respectively. The venous conduit works like an artery, bringing the blood from above downwards, unlike its earlier function of reaching blood from below up. The shorter vein grafts have higher flow rates and possibly a better long-term patency. Hence, wherever possible, the popliteal artery should be chosen as a donor artery instead of the femoral. Occasionally, even the radial artery can be used as a conduit for short segment bypasses like, the popliteo-tibial and tibio-tibial. In proximal segment block, e.g. superficial femoral, a femoro-femoral or femoro-popliteal vascular bypass is performed. In such proximal vascular bypass surgeries, a synthetic graft like, Polytetrafluoroethylene (PTFE, Gortex) can also be used as conduit (Fig. 37.9). However, diabetics frequently require bypass from femoral or popliteal to the small muscular arteries like tibial, peroneal, and dorsalis pedis for limb salvage. A good DSA is critical to determine which of these vessels are patent and in communication with the plantar vessels. The size of the vessel, the amount of occlusion, and the runoff into foot usually determine the site of distal anastomosis (recipient artery).

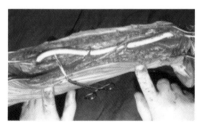

Fig. 37.9: Synthetic graft (gortex) used for femoro-femoral bypass

It is important to realise that the rate of limb salvage is typically higher than the graft patency, after an infrapopliteal bypass. Many diabetic patients have a marginal perfusion in an otherwise normal appearing foot. A minor trauma can damage the skin and can lead to a non-healing ulcer or an infection because of reduced blood supply. These ulcerations may progress and ultimately destroy the foot, thereby requiring an amputation. A revascularization of the leg can promote healing of the ulcer and restore the foot viability (Fig. 37.10 A to 37.10 D), thereby, salvaging the foot, although the graft itself might thrombose later. The increased use of lower extremity vascular re-construction has resulted in a significant decline in the incidence of amputations at all levels. The results

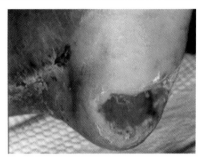

Fig. 37.10A: *Subplantar abscess and a deep calcaneal lesion

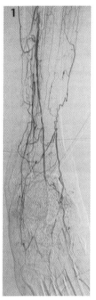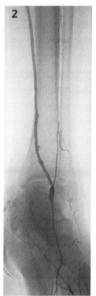

Fig. 37.10B: *Angiography showed multiple occlusions

Fig. 37.10C: *Because of the nonhealing defect, a popliteal-pedal bypass was performed

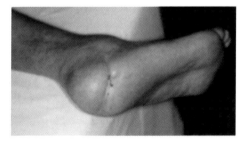

Fig. 37.10D: *Secondarily healed defect after reconstructive revascularization

of vascular reconstructions are as gratifying in diabetics as in nondiabetics. Therefore, the message to carry home is, before any major amputation in a neuro-ischemic foot in diabetics is planned a vascular surgeon must be consulted.

*Reproduced by kind permission by the International Working Group on the Diabetic Foot

MANAGEMENT OF NEUROISCHEMIC ULCER

In neuroischemic foot the blood circulation is compromised and even a trivial trauma like, shoe bite or nail injury may lead to a nonhealing ischemic ulcer, because of poor perfusion. Such ulcers are commonly seen on margins of toes or interdigital spaces. Ischemic ulcers need to be identified and aggressively treated with total rest to the foot (to minimize requirement of perfusion). Superficial eschar should be removed and ulcer should be cleaned and dressed with a non occlusive dressing.

Medical treatment should focus on intensified insulin therapy for good glycemic control, broad spectrum parentral antibiotics to prevent secondary infection, and antiplatelet agents (Aspirin, clopidogrel), hemorrheologic agents (pentoxifylline), and anticoagulants (low molecular weight heparin) should be given. If the ulcer is infected, drainage of the deep space infection is necessary. Such an infected ischemic lesion can otherwise progress rapidly and ultimately destroy the foot, leading to wet gangrene, requiring a major amputation.

Urgent evaluation of vascular status of the affected limb should be done using duplex Doppler, followed by a DSA. Multidisciplinary team involving interventional radiologist and a vascular surgeon, should plan appropriate strategy to improve circulation and foot perfusion. Whenever feasible vascular reconstruction, either by angioplasty or bypass surgery, should be planned. If vascular reconstruction is not feasible, medical management should be continued to promote natural healing of the ulcer, amputation being the last option.

MANAGEMENT OF GANGRENE

It is the end point of neuroischemic foot and is usually associated with a grave prognosis. Black discoloration of the skin is like the tip of an iceberg. There is often a significant necrosis of deeper tissues. The damage is irreversible and some form of amputation is inevitable. Medical treatment remains the same as that for a neuroischemic ulcer. Although difficult, every attempt should be made to convert wet gangrene to dry gangrene, by strict bed rest and control of infection. Evaluation of the vascular status of the affected limb and a possibility of vascular reconstruction should be explored. However, if gangrene is extensive, wet,

malodorous, and vascular reconstruction is not possible, a decision to carryout leg amputation, either above knee or below knee depending upon the vascular status, should be implemented. Hyperbaric oxygen therapy (HBO) can be tried as an adjunct to the medical and surgical treatment. HBO therapy increases tissue oxygen tension and has been advocated in advanced ischemic foot lesions.

If the gangrene is dry and limited to toes or distal foot, one can wait for mummification to occur and allow autoamputation to take place (Fig. 37.11). Vascular reconstruction, if possible, can be offered at a later date.

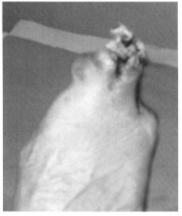

Fig. 37.11: Previous surgical amputations for 1st and 5th toes, existing lesser toes have dry gangrene and are falling off (auto amputation)

Acute Ischemia

In patients presenting with acute ischemia (Fig. 37.12), a thrombolytic therapy (urokinase) as described earlier, should be instituted and may be followed by

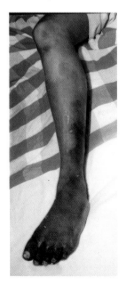

Fig. 37.12: Presentation of acute ischemia, slaty grey discoloration of toes, signs of ischemia visible upto the knee

balloon angioplasty. However, if the cause of acute ischemia is embolization, then an emergency embolectomy should be carried out (Fig. 37.13). The results are rewarding, it restores the leg perfusion immediately, and the patient's symptoms are relieved. Appropriate measures to prevent recurrence of embolization need to be taken.

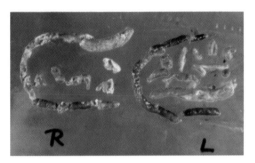

Fig. 37.13: Emboli removed from both legs in a patient with acute critical leg ischemia, emergency embolectomy led to dramatic improvement in symptoms and vascular supply to legs

SUMMARY

The management of a neuroischemic foot is difficult as compared to that of a neuropathic foot. Evaluation of the vascular status and a possibility of vascular reconstruction must be explored. Once the stage of gangrene sets in, the overall prognosis is grave. Results after leg amputation are also not satisfactory. Contralateral amputation is required in 50% in a couple of years, five year survival is less than 50% after amputation and rehabilitation is far from ideal. Early diagnosis and prompt treatment are the best ways to reduce the terrible sufferings of the patients with peripheral vascular disease.

Case Study (37.A)

This 72 year old male with type 2 DM of 8 years duration, hypertensive since 6 years and an ex-smoker, presented with severe rest pain (since 6 weeks) and discoloration of left foot 4th toe since 2 weeks. On examination, he looked anxious, his pulse rate was 110/min, BP 160/90 mmHg. His respiratory examination revealed diminished air entry and rhonchi; the other systemic examinations were normal. Lower limb examination showed palpable left femoral pulsations and absent popliteal, posterior tibial, and

dorsalis pedis pulsations. The femoral and popliteal were palpable on the right, however posterior tibial and dorsalis pedis pulsations were absent. He had loss of protective sensations and the ABI was not recordable on both sides. There was a black discoloration of the 4th toe of the left foot, without evidence of any ulceration or infection (Fig. 37.14 A).

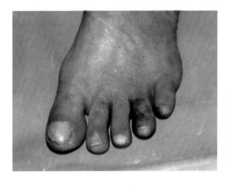

Fig. 37.14A: Black discoloration of the 4th toe in patient with chronic critical leg ischemia left

He was hospitalized and evaluated. His CBC and serum creatinine levels were normal, plasma glucose was 212 mg% and HbA1c 7.4%. His ECG showed T wave inversion in lateral leads ($V_5 V_6$), the X-ray chest showed chronic obstructive airway disease, 2-dimensional echocardiography showed diastolic dysfunction and left ventricular ejection fraction of 55%. Duplex arterial Doppler both legs revealed, atherosclerotic lesions in the superficial femoral artery, more marked on left side, with occlusive disease in the infrapopliteal vessels. Angiography of left lower limb arteries revealed diffuse occlusive disease in the superficial femoral artery with total occlusion in the lower part and evidence of partial filling of popliteal through collaterals (Fig. 37.14 B).

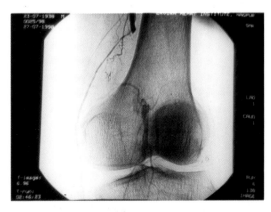

Fig. 37.14B: Angiography showing total occlusion in the lower part of superficial femoral artery

In view of critical leg ischemia, the patient underwent transluminal balloon dilatation angioplasty. The postangioplasty angiogram showed opening up of the occluded vessel (Fig. 37.14 C). The patient had partial relief in the rest pain, however, within two days

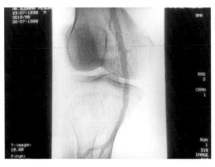

Fig. 37.14C: Postangioplasty, the vessel has reopened

it recurred. Finally, a decision to carry out bypass surgery was undertaken. Femoral artery was the donor artery and posterior tibial the recipient artery. The conduit used was reversed saphenous vein (Fig. 37.15 A, 37.15 B). There was immediate symptomatic relief, the gangrenous 4th toe gradually mummified (Fig. 37.15 C) and fell off in two months (autoamputation).

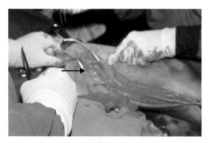

Fig. 37.15A: Reversed saphenous vein graft anastomosed to femoral (donor) artery

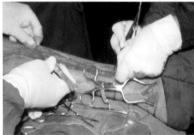

Fig. 37.15B: Site of anastomosis with posterior tibial (recipient) artery

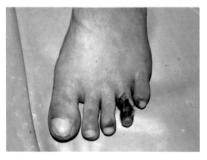

Fig. 37.15C: Mummified 4th toe left foot

This patient with critical leg ischemia and gangrene of the 4th toe, underwent balloon dilatation angioplasty with reopening of the occluded vessel, however the symptoms recurred within two days, suggesting angioplasty failure. He underwent a femoro-posterior tibial bypass surgery with a reversed saphenous venous graft with a remarkable improvement in the symptoms. He was last seen two years ago, three years after the surgery and was doing well.

Case Study (37.B)

This 64 year old male with type 2 DM of 11 years duration, presented with severe rest pain and non healing ulcers in right lower limb. His general physical and systemic examinations were normal, with a BP of 130/80 mmHg. The right lower limb examination revealed palpable femoral artery pulsations and absent popliteal with feeble posterior tibial and dorsalis pedis pulsations. The ABI was 0.5 on right side and 0.9 on left side. All the arterial pulses on left side were well felt. He had an ischemic ulcer on the dorsum of right foot and another on the anterior part of right lower leg (Fig. 37.16 A).

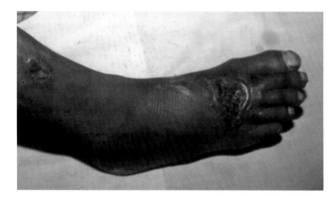

Fig. 37.16A: Ischemic ulcer on dorsum and anterior part of right lower leg

He was hospitalized and switched on to broad spectrum I/V antibiotics and intensified insulin therapy. The investigations revealed Hb 12 gms%, TLC 8100/cu.mm, ESR 38 mm/1st hr, S. creatinine 1.1 mg/dL, plasma glucose 222 mg% and HbA$_1$c 7.6%. He was subjected to right femoral angiography, which showed a complete occlusion of the superficial femoral artery from its origin. There was distal run-off in posterior tibial and dorsalis pedis, through collaterals (Fig. 37.16 B, 37.16 C).

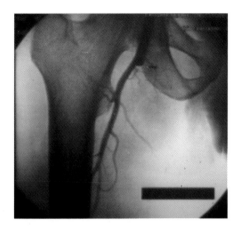

Fig. 37.16B: Angiography showing total occlusion of superficial femoral artery at its origin

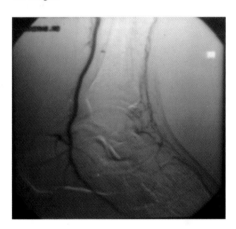

Fig. 37.16C: Angiography showing distal run-off in the posterior tibial artery through collaterals

In view of critical leg ischemia and the nonhealing ischemic ulcers, the patient was posted for femoro-posterior tibial bypass. The conduit used was saphenous vein "in situ". The proximal end of the saphenous vein was anastomosed with the femoral artery (donor artery) and the distal end with the

posterior tibial artery (recipient artery), in the middle third of the leg (Fig. 37.16 D).

The patient had a remarkable improvement in the rest pain and the ulcers showed signs of healing (Fig. 37.16 E).This patient with critical leg ischemia and ischemic ulcers had a long segment occlusion of the superficial femoral artery from its origin. Hence, femoro-posterior tibial bypass surgery, with saphenous vein graft "in situ", was performed. The

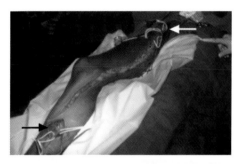

Fig. 37.16D: Intra-operative photograph showing sites of anastomosis, proximally femoral, distally posterior tibial in the middle part of the leg, saphenous vein "in situ" been used as a graft

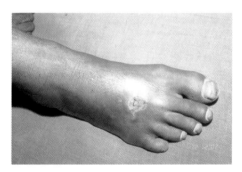

Fig. 37.16E: Ischemic ulcer healing after sucessful revascularization surgery

risk of thrombosis of venous graft "in situ" is less because of better size match. The posterior tibial artery was chosen as a recipient artery as angiography had shown distal run-off in it.

Section Six

Amputation

- Gravity of the Problem of Leg Amputation

- Minor and Major Amputations

- Rehabilitation of the Amputee

38 Gravity of the Problem of Leg Amputation

Missed only when lost

Lower limb amputation is the most devastating and tragic incident in the life of a diabetic. It leads to great suffering, prolonged hospitalization and great expense to both the patient and the community. It compromises the quality of life and leaves a demoralizing impact on the entire family.

One Amputation Every 10th minute

Diabetes is the leading cause of nontraumatic amputations. In USA it is estimated that approximately 85000 lower extremity amputations (LEA), are performed every year, which is almost one every 10th minute. In India, rough estimates indicate that approximately 45000 LEA are performed every year.

Risk of Amputation

The risk of an amputation in diabetics increases with age, duration of diabetes and male sex. The ratio of leg versus toe amputation increases significantly above the age of 65 years. LEA rate in diabetics has been reported to be the highest in Pima Indians and lowest among Asians. Premature death from coronary artery disease has been postulated to be one of the explanations for the lower rate in Asians. Overall, diabetics have a 15 times higher risk of leg amputation than non diabetic individuals.

Financial Burden

Economic considerations are an increasing concern for everyone involved in diabetes healthcare. While the exact direct and indirect costs are difficult to ascertain, the cost incurred for a major amputation in diabetics is enormous. In the western world it varies between US $ 10,000 to 25,000, whereas in India the cost ranges between US $ 1000 to 2000.

Ipsilateral and Contralateral Amputations

In diabetic patients who have undergone an amputation, the risk of ipsilateral reamputation (at a higher level) is 8 to 22% of the survivors. The risk of contralateral limb amputation increases and is 10% at one year, 23 to 30% at three years, and 28 to 51% at five years.

Mortality after Amputation

The cause of death among amputees is rarely attributed to the amputation, and is usually related to concurrent comorbid conditions such as cardiac and renal disease. Perioperative mortality is about 10% and it steadily increases with the increasing age of the patient. The 1year mortality rate in diabetic amputees ranges between 13 to 40%, three year mortality rate between 35 to 65% and the five year mortality rate between 39 to 80%.

Prevention of Amputation

It has to be realized that 85% of amputations are preceded by an ulcer. If the foot ulcers are properly managed, majority of leg amputations would be preventable. In 1989, St. Vincent Declaration announced a primary objective to reduce the rate of diabetes related amputations by at least half within five years. Many European and American centers have reported a decline in leg amputations among diabetics by more than 50%. These gratifying results have been achieved because of two factors, one, development of a team approach (education to treatment) and the advancement in vascular reconstruction (angioplasty and bypass). However in some centers of Europe, reduction in the number of leg amputations has not been achieved in the last ten years. At our center, despite our best efforts, we have not been able achieve any reduction in the number of limb amputations among our patients. This is possibly because, being a referral center, more advanced diabetic foot cases are seen where foot salvage is not possible. Although our number of amputations are on a rise, the limb amputation rate has remained steady and is about 3.5%.

As a global strategy, with particular emphasis to the developing world, it is important to develop a multidisciplinary team (footcare team) at every diabetes care center and popularize lower limb vascular reconstruction. One of the reasons why lower limb vascular reconstruction takes a backseat is that the vascular surgeons are busy operating on the coronary vessels, obviously because it is more rewarding and less time consuming.

India has a dubious distinction of being the country with highest population of diabetic patients (25 million). Here majority of leg amputations are performed in neuropathic feet with severe infection, which are potentially preventable. Unless urgent steps are taken towards prevention of diabetic foot lesions, it will not be an exaggeration to state that India might emerge as the country with highest number of leg amputations in diabetics, performed every year.

39 Minor and Major Amputations

The surgery, every surgeon hates to perform

An amputation is the most devastating and demoralizing surgery for any patient, a diabetic being no exception. Unfortunately it has to be performed 15 times more frequently in the diabetics than non-diabetics.

PRINCIPLES OF AMPUTATION

- Any amputation must be carried out above the level of gangrenous tissue.
- The residual stump should have adequate soft tissue covering consisting of skin, subcutaneous tissue and muscles. The covering of soft tissue should move freely over the enclosed bone to absorb shear forces.
- A proper contouring and bevelling of the cut bone shaft is important to prevent damage of the overlying soft tissue from within.
- A retention of a full range of proximal joint motion.
- An effort should be made to retain maximum length of residual limb to facilitate use of any future prosthesis and to reduce the energy expenditure.
- In forefoot amputations, the lever length should be preserved whenever possible, to maintain stability of the foot and normalcy of gait pattern.

Amputations are classified, as per the international consensus on diabetic foot, into minor amputations (mid tarsal or below) and major amputations (above the mid tarsal level). Various amputations carried out on lower extremity are

MINOR AMPUTATIONS (Midtarsal or Below)

- Toe disarticulation
- Ray amputation
- Transmetatarsal amputation
- Tarso-metatarsal disarticulation (Lisfranc)
- Midtarsal disarticulation (Chopart)

MAJOR AMPUTATIONS (Above Midtarsal Level)

- Ankle disarticulation (Syme)
- Transtibial amputation (below knee)
- Knee disarticulation
- Transfemoral amputation (above knee)
- Hip disarticulation

As the proximal foot amputations leave a patient severely handicapped, I feel that the minor amputations should be transmetatarsal and below and those proximal to transmetatarsal should be major amputations.

Toe Disarticulation

A toe disarticulation is the commonest amputation carried out in diabetics. The toe can be disarticulated at interphalangeal or metatarsophalangeal levels. In the diabetic foot infections, the toe is commonly disarticulated at MTP level. Usually more than one toe has to be disarticulated especially in a web space infection. In majority of the cases, an open amputation is carried out (i.e. the wound is left open) where debridement of all necrotic and infected tissue, including bone, is carried out and visually uninvolved tissue like any residual skin is preserved for the future reconstruction and closure of the wound (Fig. 39.1 to 39.3). The wound is closed at a later date, when it is absolutely free from the infection. In the forefoot infections, disarticulating a toe gives the surgeon a better opportunity to drain pus pockets and debride the necrotic tissue. One can therefore be generous with toe disarticulation, but a miser with a leg amputation.

Disarticulation of the second toe, removes lateral support to great toe resulting in a hallux valgus deformity, toe spacers can prevent it (Fig. 39.6). An isolated toe, where the toes on either side of it have been disarticulated, is functionally useless and more

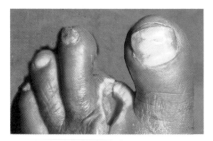

Fig. 39.1: 2nd toe disarticulation left foot (open amputation)

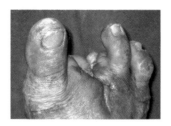

Fig. 39.2: Disarticulation of 2nd and 3rd toes, wound sutured at a later date with residual skin

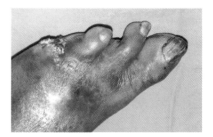

Fig. 39.3: Disarticulation of 3rd and 5th toes left foot

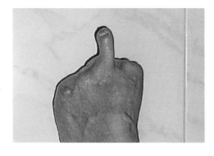

Fig. 39.4: Disarticulation of 1st, 3rd, 4th and 5th toes left foot, 2nd toe isolated, such an isolated lesser toe without any support from either side is more vulnerable for trauma and should be disarticulated as well

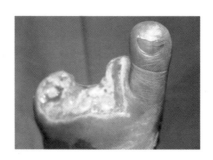

Fig. 39.5: Disarticulation of all the four lesser toes left foot, great toe preserved for better foot stability

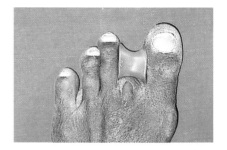

Fig. 39.6: Toe spacer to prevent hallux valgus and varus deformities of lesser toes

susceptible to injury, and is best disarticulated with the others (Fig. 39.4). However, an isolated great toe gives more stability to the foot and hence every attempt should be made to preserve it (Fig. 39.5).

Great Toe Disarticulation

In patients with osteomyelitis of the distal phalanx of the great toe, interphalangeal (IP) disarticulation should be preferred. A sufficient viable skin should

be preserved to permit closure of the wound. Preserving the proximal phalanx gives better stability to foot (Fig. 39.7). In patients with osteomyelitis involving distal and proximal phalanges, it is preferable to remove both the phalanges and necrotic tissue and preserve the plantar and dorsal skin if viable. It is better to have a boneless great toe than not to have one at all (Fig. 39.8 A, B). However, if the great toe is grossly infected, it is preferable to carry out disarticulation at MTP joint (Fig. 39.9).

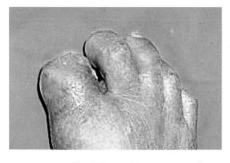

Fig. 39.7: Partial great toe amputation at IP joint right foot

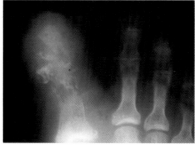

Fig. 39.8A: Osteomyelitis of proximal and distal phalanges of right great toe

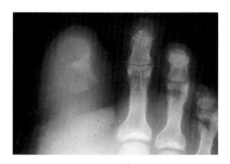

Fig. 39.8B: Infected phalanges removed, preserving dorsal and plantar skin (Boneless great toe)

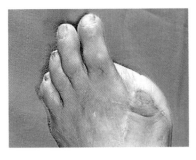

Fig. 39.9: Great toe disarticulation at 1st MTP joint

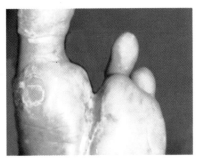

Fig. 39.13: 2nd and 3rd ray amputations left foot

Ray Amputation

A ray amputation consists of an excision of the toe and its metatarsal. A single or multiple ray resections may be required depending upon the severity of forefoot infection. As regards the first (medial) ray, a proximal shaft of the metatarsal should be preserved to preserve the medial arch of the foot (Fig. 39.10). Single ray resection of lesser rays does not affect the stability of the foot significantly (Fig. 39.11, 39.12). Multiple ray resections may be performed provided the first ray is preserved, so as to give a better stability to the foot (Fig. 39.13, 39.14A, B).

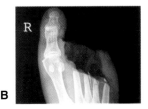

A   **B**

Fig. 39.14A and B: **(A)** Lateral 4 rays excised in an oblique fashion, 1st ray preserved for better stability of the foot, **(B)** Radiograph right foot showing partial ray amputations of lateral 4 rays in an oblique manner

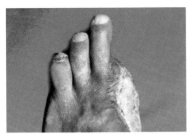

Fig. 39.10: Left 2nd toe disarticulation and 1st ray amputation, proximal part of 1st metatarsal preserved for better stability of the foot

Transmetatarsal Amputation

It is a viable option where whole of the distal forefoot is involved or the forefoot infection has involved first and second metatarsal bones. In a neuroischemic foot, it is indicated in the presence of gangrene of the distal foot, where a bypass surgery has restored the blood supply to rest of the foot.

A transmetatarsal amputation leaves a good functioning and stable foot because of a better lever length (Fig. 39.15). The metatarsal shafts should be bevelled on plantar aspect to reduce the peak plantar

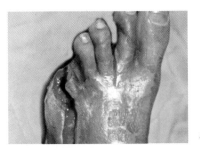

Fig. 39.11: 5th ray amputation of left foot

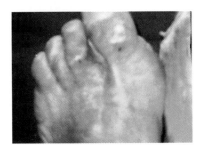

Fig. 39.12: Healed 2nd ray amputation left foot

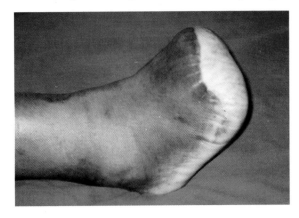

Fig. 39.15: Transmetatarsal amputation right foot, note thick plantar skin mobilized to cover the metatarsal shafts

pressure. It is essential to preserve the plantar skin to cover metatarsal shafts, the residual skin defect on the dorsum can always be covered with split skin grafts (Fig. 39.16). A plaster cast should be given to prevent equinus deformity. Once the wound has healed, the patient can wear a normal sized shoe with a filler distally.

Tarsometatarsal (Lisfranc) Disarticulation

It is indicated in severe diabetic foot infection with a preserved heel pad. This disarticulation is at the tarso metatarsal junction. The foot is severely shortened with loss of forefoot lever length (Fig. 39.17). A plaster cast should be given to prevent equinus deformity. The functioning of the foot is significantly compromised and a prosthesis is essential for limited walking.

Midtarsal (Chopart) Disarticulation

It is indicated in severe foot infection, which has progressed more proximally with preserved heel pad (Fig. 39.18). A midtarsal disarticulation is through the talo-navicular and calcaneo-cuboid joints, leaving only the hind foot (talus and calcaneus) behind. As the heel pad is preserved, the patient may do a limited walking, a prosthesis would facilitate it further.

Among the midfoot amputations (Fig. 39.19), transmetatarsal amputation leaves better functioning residual foot. Lisfranc and Chopart amputations are rarely performed in diabetic foot infections, due to an increased risk of failure and the proximity of the infected tissue to the heel pad.

Ankle Disarticulation (Syme)

It is indicated in severe diabetic foot infection, where more distal amputations are not feasible and in Charcot foot associated with severe destruction of the calcaneus.

The disarticulation is through the ankle joint with preservation of the heel flap to permit weight bearing on the end of the stump (Fig. 39.20). It is extremely important to ensure a patency of the posterior tibial artery (duplex Doppler) prior to surgery, as it is the main source of blood supply for the heel flap. It is also important to ensure that the heel pad is infection free. There is a significant functional loss after ankle disarticulation leaving the patient severely handicapped. A good training and proper prosthesis is essential (Fig. 39.21).

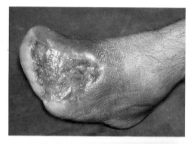
Fig. 39.16: Transmetatarsal amputation right foot, note plantar skin covering metatarsal shafts, dorsal skin defect covered by skin grafting

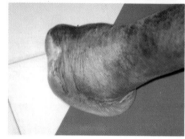
Fig. 39.17: Tarsometatarsal (Lisfranc) disarticulation

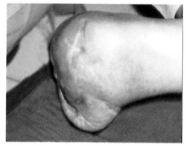
Fig. 39.18: Midtarsal (Chopart) disarticulation

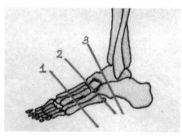
Fig. 39.19: Showing levels of midfoot amputations 1) Transmetatarsal, 2) Tarsometatarsal (Lisfranc), 3) Midtarsal (Chopart) disarticulation

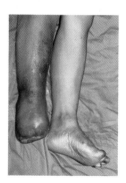
Fig. 39.20: Ankle disarticulation (Syme) right foot, left foot, toe amputation

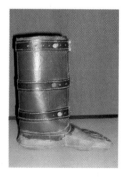
Fig. 39.21: Prosthesis after Syme's disarticulation, foot made of vulcanized rubber (Jaipur foot) and socket cushioned from inside to accomodate the stump

Transtibial (Below Knee BK) Amputation

It is indicated in:
- An advanced diabetic foot infections, which have involved the hind foot, and more distal amputations are not feasible.
- Acutely ill patient, where advanced diabetic foot infection is posing a life threatening situation.
- Charcot foot associated with severe bone destruction with infected mid foot ulceration or a flail ankle, which has made walking impossible.
- A neuroischemic foot where a vascular reconstruction for foot salvage is not feasible.

Among the major amputations performed for a diabetic foot, BK amputation is the commonest. The site of amputation is usually at the junction of the proximal two thirds and distal one third of the leg (Fig. 39.22, 39.23), although a shorter stump is also possible. The longer stump requires less energy to walk and has a good artificial limb prosthesis function. The greatest advantage of BK amputation is that the knee joint is preserved, making rehabilitation with a prosthetic limb successful in the majority. In fact, one cannot make out the physical handicap of the patient from a distance. The patients with artificial limb can walk, run, climb, and ride bicycle efficiently. At every clinic visit however, the stump should be examined for callosities and friction injuries.

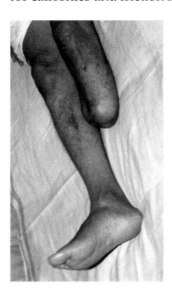 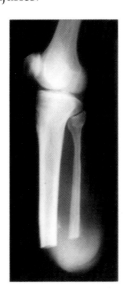

Fig. 39.22: BK amputation left, note adequate length of the residual limb

Fig. 39.23: Radiograph showing stump after BK amputation, note adequate soft tissue covering over resected bone shafts

Knee Disarticulation

It is indicated in:
- Diabetic foot infection which has extended above the ankle and primary healing of the stump of B K amputation is doubtful.
- In a neuroischemic foot, where a vascular reconstruction for limb salvage is not feasible and the infrapopliteal disease is likely to pose a threat to primary stump healing of BK amputation.

Although it is believed that a knee disarticulation is the next best level after a BK amputation, as compared to an AK amputation, it is rerely performed. A knee disarticulation is simpler, associated with less blood loss and a rapid postoperative recovery because virtually no muscle tissue is transected (Fig. 39.24). There is greater bed mobility and sitting balance as compared to an AK amputation. I recollect having seen a knee disarticulation being performed only in one patient who had necrotizing fascitis.

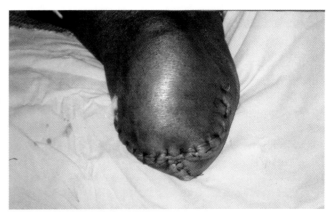

Fig. 39.24: Right knee disarticulation

Transfemoral (Above Knee, AK) Amputation

It is indicated in:
- Severe diabetic foot infection which has extended in the leg and even knee disarticulation is not feasible.
- A neuroischemic foot with an extensive gangrene or a critical leg ischemia where neither vascular reconstruction nor a BK amputation are feasible. An AK amputation is commonly performed in advanced peripheral vascular disease, in old patients, bed ridden patients, and in patients who have a multi system involvement.

The stump should be as long as possible that can be adequately covered with muscles and skin to minimize the excess energy expenditure. The femur is usually divided 4 to 5 inches (10-12 cm) above the knee joint (Fig. 39.25 A, B). The energy expenditure after AK amputations is increased significantly and very few diabetic patients can really become ambulatory after the surgery.

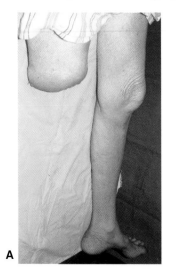 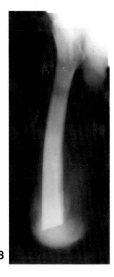

Fig. 39.25A and B: **(A)** Right AK amputation, note adequate length of the residual limb, **(B)** Radiograph of the same patient, note the stump been adequately covered with soft tissue

Hip Disarticulation

It is indicated in a fulminant diabetic foot infection, where an A K amputation is not feasible and the patient is critically ill. The major vessels like the femoral artery and vein are ligated and the femoral and sciatic nerves are divided. All the major muscles with their attachments on the femur are dissected. The hip joint capsule and ligamentum teres are incised and the hip disarticulation is completed. A hip disarticulation is in the true sense, a complete lower extremity amputation. I recollect having seen only one hip disarticulation, which was carried out for an advanced necrotizing fascitis, the patient succumbed within a few days of surgery.

Risk of Contralateral Amputation

After a B K amputation, the work of walking (energy expenditure) increases and the amputees decrease their walking speed in order to maintain the rate of oxygen uptake. A K amputees have both decreased walking speed and increased rate of oxygen uptake. The extra weight-bearing load placed on the remaining

extremity increases the risk of contra-lateral foot ulceration, which may eventually progress to contra-lateral amputation (Fig. 39.26, 39.27).

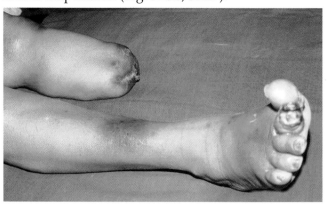

Fig. 39.26: Left BK amputation, right infected 2nd toe with necrosis

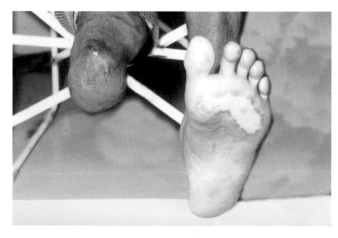

Fig. 39.27: Right BK amputation, left healed plantar wound, depigmented area indicating thermal injury

PVD in diabetics is invariably bilateral. Once the patient with a neuro-ischemic foot undergoes a major amputation, the risk of contralateral amputation in increased significantly to a tune of 50% in 5 years. The rehabilitation becomes further difficult and the quality of life becomes miserable. Most of these patients are old, disabled and spend the rest of their lives in bed. The mortality after a contralateral amputation can be as high as 50% in five years.

Trauma and diabetes are the two commonest indications for amputations in the lower limb. However, there are significant clinical differences between these two conditions, which impact on the results, morbidity, and mortality after surgery. The patients with trauma are often young, otherwise healthy, the foot is injured but not infected and they have an intact peripheral nervous as well as vascular systems, unlike their diabetic counterparts. Various amputations like tarso-metatarsal, mid-tarsal, ankle disarticulation were originally described for trauma cases and later applied to the diabetic foot.

In my opinion, of all the amputations described for the lower limb in diabetics, toe disarticulation, ray, transmetalarsal, B K, and A K amputations are more definitive and yield the best possible results. Amputations like tarso-metatarsal, mid-tarsal, and ankle disarticulation are associated with several problems like recurrent ulcerations, foot deformities, and difficulties with prostheses and functioning of the foot. Many a time I feel that patients after below knee amputation do much better functionally, and their quality of life is far better than some of those who have undergone proximal foot amputations.

Case Study (39.A)

I recollect an 82 years old man, father of a doctor, with longstanding type 2 DM, renal failure and severe bilateral air to iliac occlusive disease. When I saw him, he had extensive gangrene of right foot, had undergone A K amputation left 3 years back, amputation of penis 2 years back and was on chronic ambulatory peritoneal dialysis. He was praying to me to save his right gangrenous foot. I could not fulfill his wishes and fortunately for me, I lost him for followup.

Case Study (39.B)

This 50 years old female with type 2 DM of 20 years duration, hypertension since 12 years, presented with non healing wound right foot since 1 month. History revealed that she had a plantar ulcer of longstanding, on the 1st MTH. This ulcer started discharging purulent material one month ago, for which she had consulted a surgeon elsewhere, who carried out great toe disarticulation at MTP joint and since the wound failed to heal, she reported to us. Her general physical examination was normal except BP 160/100 mmHg. Her systemic examination was normal. She had neuropathic feet with normal ABI. The right foot showed an infected ulcer at the site of 1st MTP joint. The ulcer had slough and necrotic tissue and discharged pus on pressure (Fig. 39.28 A). The investigations revealed Hb 7.5 gms%, TLC 9700/cu.mm, ESR 110 mm/1st hr, plasma glucose 328 mg%

and HbA$_1$c 9.8%. The X-ray revealed destruction of 1st MTH and osteomyelitis of metatarsal shaft. She was hospitalized, switched on to multiple injections of insulin, intravenous antibiotics and posted for surgery. She underwent **1st ray amputation** and debridement of the slough and necrotic tissue. After three weeks of regular dressings, the wound granulated (Fig. 39.28 B). Two weeks later the wound had shrunk and was then covered with a split skin graft (Fig. 39.28 C). The patient was given protective footwear and necessary instructions for proper foot care.

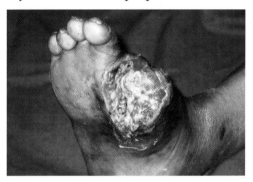

Fig. 39.28A: Right foot ulcer, after 1st MTP disarticulation, note necrotic areas and slough

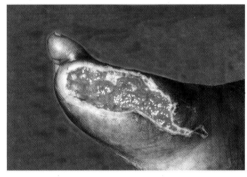

Fig. 39.28B: After 1st ray amputation, wound granulating

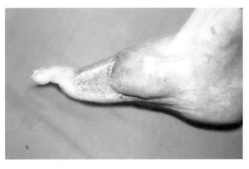

Fig. 39.28C: After skin grafting, note medial arch preserved, because the proximal portion of 1st metatarsal was retained

Case Study (39.C)

The 48 years old male with type 2 DM of five years duration, presented with swelling and non healing wound left foot since six weeks, which had developed after a stone prick. His general physical and systemic examinations were normal. He had neuropathic feet with normal ABI. Examination of left foot revealed cellulitis, deep ulceration over the dorsum with destruction of deep tissues with purulent discharge. Plantar aspect revealed erythematous midfoot swelling extending upto 2nd and 3rd toes. His investigations revealed Hb 9.5 gms%, TLC 9800/cu.mm, ESR 130 mm/1st hr, S. Creatinine 1.5 mg/dL, and plasma glucose 389 mg% and HbA$_1$c 10.4%. X-ray left foot revealed osteomyelitis of all the phalanges of 2nd and 3rd toes and involvement of the 2nd and 3rd MTP joints. He was hospitalized, switched on to broad spectrum intravenous antibiotics, multiple injections of insulin and was posted for surgical debridement. He underwent **2nd and 3rd ray amputations** with debridement of necrotic material. His foot was practically divided (Fig. 39.29 A, 39.29 B) in the centre and both dorsal and plantar wounds regularly debrided and dressed. Four weeks later, he underwent split skin grafting for both wounds simultaneously (Fig. 39.29 C). The patient is being regularly followed up since last 8 years. Although his foot has been salva-

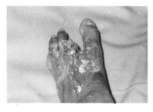

Fig. 39.29A: Dorsal view left after 2nd and 3rd ray amputations

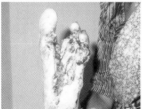

Fig. 39.29B: Plantar view, note left foot been practically divided in the centre

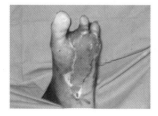

Fig. 39.29C: After skin grafting

ged, he has developed hallux valgus deformity and varus deformities of lateral 2 toes. The plantar skin graft has contracted and has a callosity over the 4th MTH due to altered biomechanics (Fig. 39.30 A, B).

The patient is using protective footwear and has been advised to minimize his activity level.

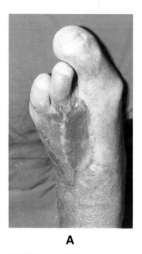 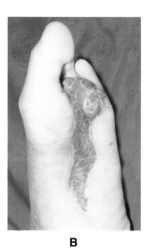

A **B**

Fig. 39.30A and B: (A) 8 yrs later, note hallux valgus and varus deformities of lesser toes, intact skin graft, **(B)** Plantar view, note hyperpigmented, contracted but intact skin graft and callosity over 4th MT head

Case Study (39.D)

This 46 years old male with type 2 DM of 10 years duration presented with nonhealing wound right foot and swelling. He was a known hypertensive since 6 years and had undergone laser photocoagulation both eyes for diabetic retinopathy. His general physical examination showed that he was obese with a BMI of 31, BP 150/96 mmHg. His systemic examination was normal. He had neuropathic feet with normal ABI. The right foot plantar aspect showed swelling, erythema and large deep necrotic ulcer over the 1st MTH extending into the ball of great toe and the 1st web space. He had another ulcer over the 4th MTH which had extended into the 3rd web space. The wound was malodorous and discharged purulent material. His investigations revealed Hb 11 gms%, TLC 9100/cumm, ESR 128 mm/1st hr, plasma glucose 450mg% and HbA$_1$c 10.2%. X-ray right foot showed osteomyelitis of the proximal phalanx of great toe with destruction of 1st MTP joint, and 4th MTH (Fig. 39.31 A). The patient was hospitalized, switched on to intravenous antibiotics, multiple injections of insulin and was posted for surgery. On exploration of the wound

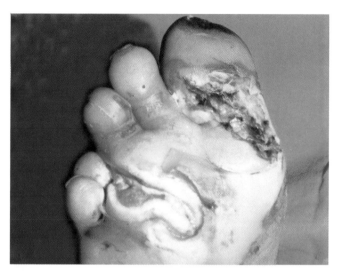

Fig. 39.31A: Grossly infected right forefoot, with deep ulcerations

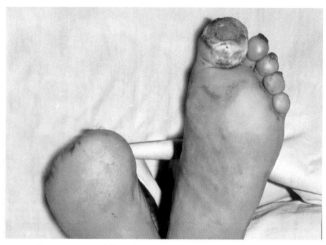

Fig. 39.32A: Ulcer on contralateral foot (great toe)

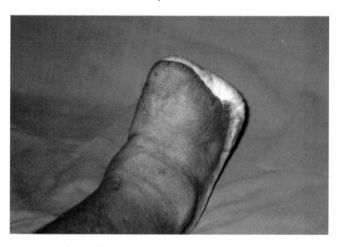

Fig. 39.31B: After transmetatarsal amputation right foot

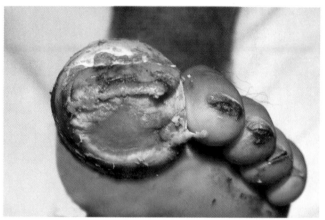

Fig. 39.32B: Great toe ulcer with necrotic margin (closer view)

it was seen that deeper tissues were grossly infected and hence **transmetatarsal amputation** was carried out (Fig. 39.31 B). The metatarsal shafts on the plantar aspect were bevelled. The plantar skin was mobilized to cover the metatarsal shafts and was sutured with the skin of the dorsum. Patient made an uneventful recovery and was given protective footwear with filler distally. **The story did not end here.**

This gentleman is a mathematics teacher and is required to stand several hours a day in the classroom. He also rode a two wheeler with a 'Kick-start', despite repeated instructions to change over to a 'self-starting' two wheeler and use a chair to sit in the classroom. However he did not pay any heed and landed up with a contralateral foot ulcer (great toe) (Fig. 39.32 A, B). The ulcer was debrided and it eventually healed in 2

months. Six months later, he presented with another ulcer over the plantar aspect of the stump (Fig. 39.33). The ulcer was deep (wagner grade 2) and was surrounded by a thick macerated callus. The callus was removed and ulcer cleaned. He was advised

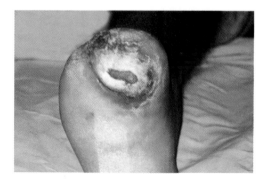

Fig. 39.33: Ulcer surrounded by thick macerated callus on the plantar aspect of the stump

antibiotics, dressings and strict non weight bearing. Our educator reinforced the importance of using of his feet sparingly. But, he returned once again! this time with a ghastly, deep heel pad infection extending between the medial and lateral borders on the plantar aspect of the heel (Fig. 39.34 A, B). His previous ulcer, over the stump, however had not deteriorated. The X-ray did not reveal osteomyelitis of the calcaneus and duplex Doppler was also normal. At this stage he was advised hospitalization and debridement, which he declined and went home. It was learnt that he underwent BK amputation, right leg, 15 days later.

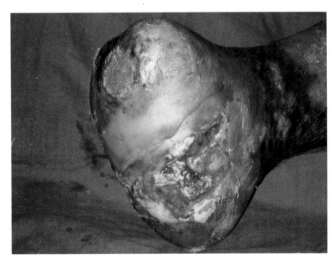

Fig. 39.34A: Deep infected ulceration on the heel pad medial view, note previous ulcer has not deteriorated

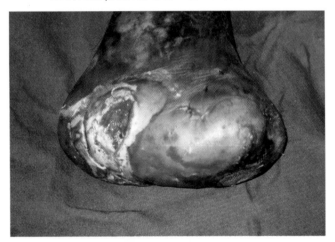

Fig. 39.34B: Deep infected ulceration on the heel pad lateral view

Non compliance and increased activity level after foot amputation, increase the risk of ulceration over both, contralateral and ipsilateral feet. This patient, at the age of 47 years, had to lose his limb because of his stubbornness. Once the foot has ulcerated, recurrence is always on the card. Frequent ulcerations, as in this case, are frustrating, both, to the patient and the treating footcare team.

Case Study (39.E)

This 80 years old male with type 2 DM of seven years, with ischemic heart disease, dilated cardiomyopathy and hypertension, presented with non healing wound over the left great toe since 3 weeks. His general physical examination revealed pulse rate of 110/min, BP 150/90 mmHg; there were no signs of cardiac failure. His cardiovascular examination revealed a systolic murmur at cardiac apex and S3 gallop. The other systemic examination was normal. He had neuropathic feet and ABI was 0.7 on both sides. His left foot showed infected wound over the great toe with cellulitis on the dorsum (Fig. 39.35 A). His investigations revealed Hb 9 gms%, TLC 9400/cu.mm, ESR 62 mm/1st hr, S. creatinine of 1.4 mg/dl, plasma glucose 244 mg% and HbA_1c 8.3%. His ECG showed old anterior wall infarction, X-ray chest showed cardiomegaly and 2-dimensional echocardiography showed ejection fraction of 30% with left ventricular wall motion abnormality. His X-ray foot revealed osteomyelitis of great toe phalanges and duplex Doppler of left lower limb arterial system showed diffuse atherosclerotic vascular disease in femoral as well as infrapopliteal vessels with biphasic waveform without any focal stenotic lesion.

Clinical diagnosis of type 2 DM, old anterior wall mycocardial infarction, hypertension, dilated cardiomyopathy with neuroischemic feet with deep tissue infection of left great toe extending into the dorsum of the foot was made. Vascular surgeon was consulted who ruled out any vascular reconstruction, in view of diffuse narrowing of the vessels and concurrent co-morbid conditions.

He was hospitalized, switched on to intravenous antibiotics, multiple injections of insulin, and medication for his cardiovascular illness were continued. In view of his compromised clinical condition, he was taken for radical debridement, of the left foot wound, under regional block anaesthesia. The great toe was disarticulated at the 1st MTP joint and necrotic skin and deep tissue over the dorsum of the foot were excised (Fig. 39.35 B). He was put on low molecular

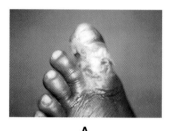 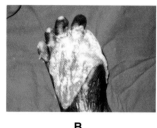 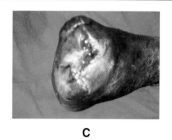 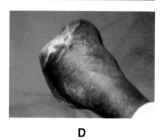

A   B   C   D

Figs 39.35A to D: (A) Infected left great toe with cellulitis, **(B)** After great toe disarticulation and debridement, **(C)** After tarsometatarsal amputation (Lisfranc) note, loosely sutured wound, **(D)** Stump healed in six weeks

weight heparine 3200 i.u. subcutaneously. Three days after the debridement, the 2nd toe showed gangrenous changes and discoloration of the 3rd and 4th toes as well, indicating, a compromised circulation. The patient was posted for more proximal amputation, i.e. **tarso-metatarsal amputation**. The wound was closed with loose sutures and it healed over 6 weeks (Fig. 39.35 C, 39.35 D). He was then given special footwear with ankle support and filler. Patient could walk and carry out simple activities and continued to remain ulcer free for 18 months, before he died suddenly after an acute episode of left ventricular failure.

Managing the diabetic foot in elderly is difficult, especially so when they have advanced systemic disease, as in this case. The surgery has to be definitive, even if it means a more proximal amputation; they cannot withstand repeated surgeries.

Case Study (39.F)

This 52 years old female with type 2 DM of 10 years duration was referred with a nonhealing wound, on right foot, since 6 weeks. History revealed that patient had a fissure over the great toe, to begin with, which got infected and progressed to marked swelling of the foot, for which she was hospitalized elsewhere. She underwent surgical debridement and partial ray amputation of the 1st 4 medial rays, leaving only the little toe. Despite debridement, the wound was malodorous and full of slough and necortic tissue (Fig. 39.36 A, 39.36 B).

The patient was hospitalized. She was switched on to broad spectrum intravenous antibiotics and intensified insulin therapy. Her general examination revealed that she was febrile, had tachycardia, was toxic and pale. Her BP was 150/90 mmHg. Her systemic examination was normal. Local examination revealed, she had a neuroischemic foot with ABI of

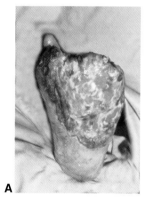 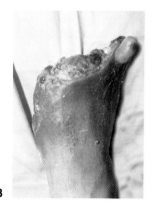

A   B

Fig. 39.36A and B: (A) At presentation, note 1st 4 rays removed, wound unhealthy with slough and necrotic tissue, **(B)** Right foot dorsal view, note isolated 5th toe and unhealthy wound

0.7 on right and 0.9 on left. Her investigations revealed Hb 7.5 gms%, TLC 14400 cu.mm, ESR 152 mm/hr, serum creatinine 0.7 mg/dL, HbA$_1$c 10.7% and plasma glucose 385 mg%. She also had background diabetic retinopathy and overt nephropathy. Her resting ECG was normal. Duplex Doppler revealed generalised narrowing in the superficial femoral artery with popliteal refilling by collaterals. A joint meeting with vascular and plastic and reconstructive surgeons, was organised. It was decided to carryout a vascular bypass with simultaneous proximal foot amputation. However, the patient was unwilling for even an angiography, leave apart a vascular bypass! At this stage, we had two options which were to either carry out a leg amputation or take a chance and salvage the foot by carrying out a proximal midfoot amputation.

Ankle systolic pressure of 104 mmHg and an ABI of 0.7, prompted us to go ahead with **midtarsal disarticulation (Chopart)**. The skin defect was later closed by a split skin graft (Fig. 39.36 C, 39.36 D). She was

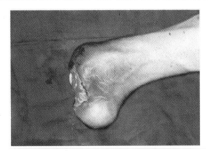

Fig. 39.36C: After midtarsal amputation (Chopart)

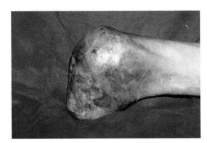

Fig. 39.36D: After skin grafting

rehabilitated and given a special boot which had the Jaipur Foot, made from vulcanized rubber, with a cushioned instep and ankle support (Fig. 39.37).

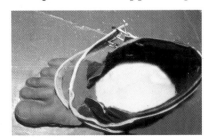

Fig. 39.37: Prosthesis, with 'Jaipur foot', with cushioned instep

In such a dysvascular, neuroischemic foot, carrying out a proximal foot amputation was a difficult proposition. Fortunately, in this patient, foot salvage was possible.

She is being regularly followed up for last 5 years (Fig. 39.38 A, 39.38 B), is able to carryout house hold activities and attend social functions too! She has been adhering to our instructions of minimal use of her feet.

Case Study (39.G)

This 68 years male with type 2 DM since 12 years, presented with non healing wound right foot, since 6 weeks, associated with swelling and fever. History revealed noticed swelling and pus discharge from the

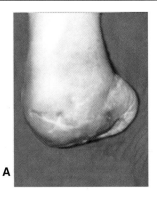
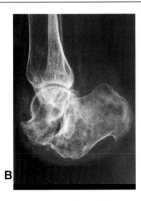

Fig. 39.38A and B: **(A)** Five years later, healed healthy stump, **(B)** Radiograph of the stump showing marked osteoporosis, due to its limited use

5th toe, 6 weeks ago, for which he was prescribed antibiotics, dressings and was advised to continue the twice a day insulin therapy. On examination, his pulse rate was 120/min, he was febrile and toxic and BP 130/80 mmHg. Local examination revealed that he had neuropathic feet and normal ABI, a swollen right foot with necrosis of the skin over 4th toe, deep interdigital ulceration and a deep ulcer medially on the 5th toe. Plantar aspect showed swelling and yellowish discoloration (Fig. 39.39 A, 39.39 B).

He was hospitalized and switched on to I/V antibiotics and metronidazole, intensified insulin therapy. His investigations revealed Hb 9.2 gms%, TLC 12800/cu.mm, ESR 139 mm/1st hr, S. creatinine 1.7 mg/dL, plasma glucose 346 mg% and HbA$_1$c 9.6. His resting ECG was normal. His X-ray foot showed osteomyelitis of the 5th toe phalanges. The duplex arterial Doppler was normal. A clinical diagnosis of deep seated lateral compartment infection with extension into the central compartment, was made.

He was subjected to a radical surgical debridement and amputations of 3 lateral rays; the necrotic tissue was debrided (Fig. 39.39 C, 39.39 D).

Despite radical debridement and ray amputations, the wound continued to discharge pus and there was no significant improvement in the patients general condition. The pus culture revealed growth of *Klebsiella and Staphylococus aureus* sensitive to cefoperazone. He was hence started on to inj. cefoperazone + sulbactum 2 gm 12 hrly and I/V metronidazole was continued. Seven days after, with no signs of improvement in the wound and the patient's general condition, a decision to carry out **below knee amputation** was taken and implemented. There was a remarkable

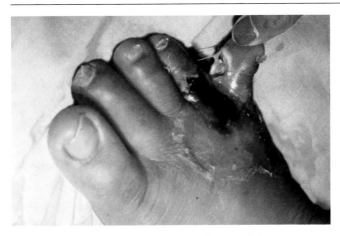

Fig. 39.39A: Right foot, 4th webspace infection, ulcer 5th toe with necrosis of the skin

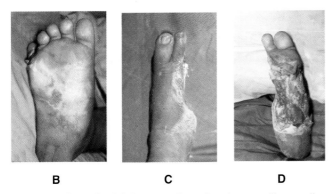

| B | C | D |

Fig. 39.39B to D: **(B)** Plantar view showing swelling, yellow discoloration indicating deep plantar infection spreading from lateral into central and medial compartments, **(C)** Dorsal view, postdebridement, amputation 3 lateral rays, **(D)** Plantar view, note extensive debridement with lateral 3 ray amputations, this patient eventually required a BK Amputation

improvement in the general health. The patient was discharged 7 days post operatively.

In this patient, the wound had begun with an ulceration of the 5th toe, which led to a further spread, osteomyelitis and extension into the lateral compartment. In the absence of a radical debridement, the infection had extended into the central compartment causing extensive foot destruction. Early surgical intervention in the form of 5th toe disarticulation and debridement, could have prevented the leg amputation.

Case Study (39.H)

This 86 year old male with type 2 DM of 22 years duration, an exsmoker, presented with black discolouration of the left foot, severe pain and hence sleepless nights despite high doses of analgesics and sedatives since one month. He had history of fracture neck femur right side, 2 years ago, which was treated conservatively, resulting in a limp. On examination, his pulse rate was 100/min, he was febrile, BP 130/80 mmHg. His respiratory system examination revealed diminished air entry on both sides and rhonchi; the other systemic examination was normal.

He was hospitalized, switched on to I/V antibiotics and intensified insulin therapy. His investigations revealed Hb 11 gms%, TLC 8600/cumm, ESR 46 mm/1st hr, S. creatinine, 1.4 mg/dL, plasma glucose 228 mg% and HbA$_1$c 7.8. Resting ECG showed old myocardial infarction. 2 D echocardiography revealed dyskinesia of the anterior wall of left ventricle, systolic and diastolic dysfunction with ejection fraction of 40%. X-ray chest revealed evidence of chronic obstructive airway disease. The duplex arterial Doppler left lower limb revealed diffuse atherosclerotic changes in superficial femoral, popliteal and also in the 3 infrapopliteal vessels.

A clinical diagnosis of type 2 DM, old myocardial infarction, left ventricular dysfunction, chronic obstructive airway disease, chronic critical leg ischemia with extensive gangrene of left foot (Fig. 39.40) and old fracture neck femur right side, was made. The vascular surgeon was consulted, who ruled out any vascular reconstruction in view of old age, associated co-morbid conditions and the physical handicap of right leg. A decision to perform **above knee amputation** was taken and executed. The patient had marked relief in pain and could enjoy some sleep with alprazolam 0.5 mg at night.

In this patient, the decision of above knee amputation instead of vascular reconstruction was taken in view of his old age and concurrent co-morbid conditions.

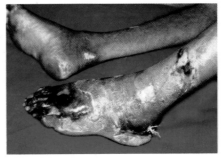

Fig. 39.40: Extensive gangrene left foot. This patient required AK amputation

40 Rehabilitation of the Amputee

After amputation, life is not normal,
But whose life is!

A rehabilitation after a major amputation is a challenging job. The overall results of rehabilitation depend upon several factors.

- Age and physical strength of the patient; older patients and debilitated patients do not do so well.
- For amputees in general, the metabolic cost of ambulation (energy expenditure) is increased and overall velocity (speed) of walking is decreased.
- Compliance and desire of the patient to become ambulatory.
- The cause of amputation. Patients with neuropathy do better than those with a peripheral vascular disease.
- Length of the stump. Greater the residual limb length, more is the improvement in ambulation.
- Type of amputation. Those with unilateral BK amputation do far better than those with a unilateral AK amputation.
- Rehabilitation of bilateral amputees is extremely difficult. An ambulation is possible if atleast one anatomical knee joint is preserved.

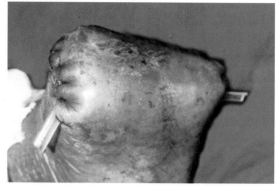

Fig. 40.1: Postoperative mid foot stump, note corrugated rubber drain

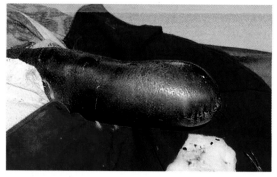

Fig. 40.2: Swollen stump after BK Amputation. Regular milking out during the dressing reduces the swelling

Postoperative Management

The goals of immediate post-surgical treatment are a reduction of edema and promotion of healing (Fig. 40.1, 40.2). The patient is trained for bed mobility, transfers to and from the wheel chair and passive exercises of the residual limb. B K amputees should avoid knee flexion for prolonged period, while AK amputees should avoid abduction by placing a pillow laterally. In addition the patient has to be trained for toilet and other day-to-day activities (Fig. 40.3). Once the wound has completely healed, the patient is trained to use crutches or a walker to promote ambulation. The patients with bilateral amputation need to be trained to use a wheelchair.

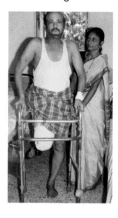

Fig. 40.3: After AK amputation, patient mobilized with a walker

Phantom Limb

The majority of amputees experience a phantom pain or phantom sensation with the passing time. These peculiar phenomena gradually disappear. The phantom pain is a painful sensation experienced with the non-existing amputated limb. The perception of pain varies from patient to patient and the type of pain varies from a dull ache to a stabbing pain. The phantom sensation, on the other hand, is a painless awareness of the nonexisting limb. The exact cause of phantom limb is however not known. It is important to reassure the amputee that these feelings are to be expected and that these would gradually decrease with time and disappear eventually. Early use of the stump with a temporary or permanent prosthesis are effective measures to overcome these problems.

Care of the Contralateral Limb

The preservation and care of the contralateral limb is of paramount importance. This limb has to compensate for the amputee's inability to maintain equal weight distribution between limbs and must accept a greater proportion of the body weight. This significantly increases the risk of foot ulceration in the contralateral limb.

Therefore, the goal of rehabilitation must include education about foot-care of contralateral limb. The patient should be made aware of the impending dangers from the onset of rehabilitation, since a high percentage will eventually lose their contralateral limb within a few years. The functional ambulation of a bilateral amputee is extremely difficult.

PROSTHESIS FOR AMPUTEES

There have been tremendous developments in the field of artificial limb prosthesis. It is beyond the scope of this atlas to discus them in depth. However few commonly used limb prostheses will be discussed. There has been a technological revolution in this field and the goal has been to make artificial limbs as functional as possible and enable the patient with artificial limb to carry out practically all the activities which he/she would with an intact limb. The whole idea is to improve the quality of life.

A prosthesis has three major parts:
• The interface consisting of the stump-socket complex

• The 'skeleton' which replaces the lost limb segments
• The artificial joints

All movements in a lower-limb prosthesis, even in those with external power, is imparted by the stump via the stump-socket interface. The design of the stump is the responsibility of the surgeon, while the prosthetist is responsible for fashioning the socket.

Jaipur foot Prosthesis

Jaipur foot prosthesis is the most economical and widely used mechanical type of prosthesis in India. It consists of a foot made up of vulcanized rubber on which a high density polythene socket is attached (Fig. 40.6). The socket is molded at high temperatures according to the shape and size of the stump. It was created by Dr. Sethi, an orthopedic surgeon from the historical city of Jaipur in Rajasthan, India and hence the name "Jaipur Foot". This prosthesis for below knee amputation allows the patients to walk, run, climb, ride a bicycle, drive vehicles, and also squat! (Fig. 40.4, 40.7). Patients can even walk barefoot when visiting religious places. The greatest advantage for its wide acceptance is its low cost, which ranges between US $ 10-40. The prosthesis for above knee amputation has a lock at the knee joint, which helps the patient to flex the limb while sitting (Fig. 40.5). However it does not allow flexion during walking. Hence, the patient has to walk with an extended limb causing a limp, which is noticeable.

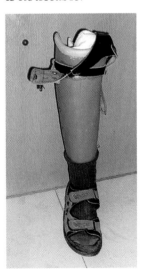

Fig. 40.4: "Jaipur foot" prosthesis for BK amputation

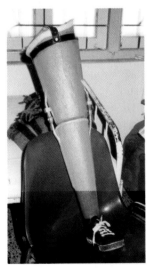

Fig. 40.5: "Jaipur foot" prosthesis for AK amputation

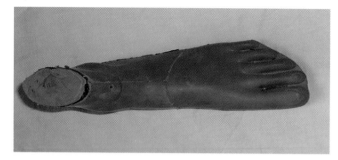

Fig. 40.6: "Jaipur foot" made of vulcanized rubber

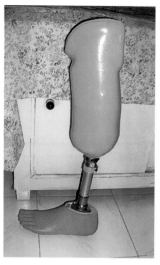

Fig. 40.8: Intelligent posthesis for BK amputation

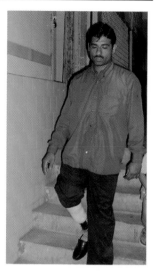

Fig. 40.9: Patient wearing endolite prosthesis right

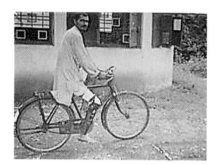

Fig. 40.7: Patient riding bicycle with BK prosthesis

Intelligent Prosthesis

The technological revolution has made it possible to create a prosthesis and foot, which can be programmed and controlled by a microelectronic control. The foot and prosthesis are made up of special metal alloys and the socket is made of endolite (Fig. 40.8 to 40.10). This prosthesis has an advantage over the conventional because of the following.

- It has more control, needs less effort by the user and is easy to maintain by the prosthetist.
- It has more precise functions, has better shock absorption and a wider range of adjustment.
- It needs micro batteries and has a pocket size programmer with coded receiver activation.
- The advantage for an above knee prosthesis is that the knee can be flexed while walking and can be programmed to match the user's style of walk, making it appear more natural.

The cost of an intelligent prosthesis ranges between us $ 500 to 5000 approximately.

Prostheses for Bilateral Amputees

The rehabilitation of these amputees is an extremely difficult proposal. The patients with bilateral below knee amputation can be given prostheses which allow

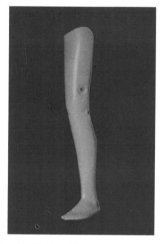

Fig. 40.10: Intelligent prosthesis for AK amputation

the patients to stand or walk a little (Fig. 40.11 A, 40.11 B). Rehabilitation in patients with bilateral above knee amputation is even more difficult and majority of these patients spend their remaining life either in the bed or a wheelchair. They are given "stubbies" to begin with and their height can be increased gradually (Fig. 40.12). Rehabilitation is comparitively easier if the patient has atleast one functional knee joint (Fig. 40.13).

Stump Care

Amputees at various levels have distinctive problems of fitting and alignment of prostheses and skin problems with the stump. Every patient should be

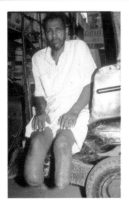 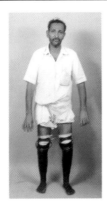

Fig. 40.11A and B: **(A)** Patient with bilateral BK amputations, **(B)** Rehabilitation with bilateral Jaipur feet prostheses

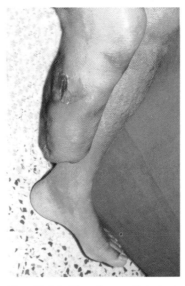

Fig. 40.14: Abrasion on the stump

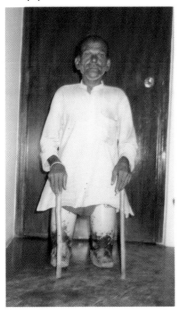

Fig. 40.12: Bilateral AK amputee been given "stubbies"

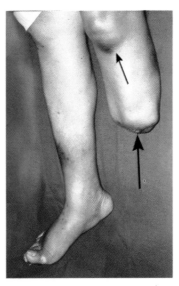

Fig. 40.15: Stump of BK amputation showing callosities (arrows), contralateral foot showing ulceration

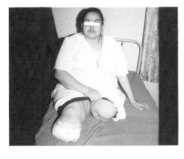

Fig. 40.13: Bilateral amputee, right BK amputation, left AK amputation, note one functional knee joint preserved

instructed to visually inspect the stump itself, as well as the contralateral foot everyday for abrasions, or ulcerations (Fig. 40.14, 40.15). The stump sock should be changed daily and replaced once it has worn out. The common stump problems are skin irritation, folliculitis, fungal infection, and ulceration. The patient should be instructed to report such problems immediately to the foot-care team. In the presence of an active ulceration at the stump, the prosthesis should not be worn until healing occurs. The common causes of skin irritation are the high pressure points within the socket. The prosthesis should be regularly checked and maintained by a prosthetist. At every clinic visit, the stump should be examined by the foot-care team.

The rehabilitation of an amputee after traumatic amputation, is different from that of a diabetic amputee. The former is usually younger, in sound health and has intact sensations and vasculature in both the residual limb as well as the contralateral limb, as against a diabetic amputee who is usually old, has multi-system involvement, loss of protective sensations, and diminished blood supply to the residual and the contralateral limb. The performance after prosthesis is therefore, not comparable in these two different settings. I know of a young South Indian classical dancer, who lost her limb (BK amputation) in an accident and within a year resumed her stage performance with an unmatched skill. The goals of rehabilitation should be appropriate to the age of the patient and his pre-amputation functional level, setting too high goals can often be counter productive.

Section Seven

Prevention of the Diabetic Foot

- Life Long Surveillance of the High-risk Feet

- Preventive Footwear

- Diabetic Foot Clinic and Team Approach

- Patient Education

41 Life Long Surveillance of the High-risk Feet

Preserve the intact skin, use the feet sparingly. The patients need to love their feet

Globally there were estimated to be approximately 135 million adults with diabetes in 1995, by the year 2025 the figure is expected to rise to 300 million. Currently, it can be presumed that the figure is around 175 million, which means there are 350 million feet which have the potential to progress to foot pathology. Several studies have shown that comprehensive footcare programmes including education, regular foot examination, identification of high risk feet, risk categorization, and longterm surveillance of high risk feet can reduce the occurrence of foot lesions in upto 50% of patients. The International consensus on the diabetic foot has identified five cornerstones for prevention:

- Regular inspection and examination of the feet and footwear.
- Identification of the high risk patient.
- Education of patient, family and healthcare providers.
- Appropriate footwear.
- Treatment of nonulcerative pathology.

IDENTIFICATION OF HIGH RISK FEET

It has to be realized that the feet should be examined at every clinic visit, the feet at high risk of ulceration need to be identified and should receive life long surveillence by the diabetes footcare team.

The two most important risk factors for foot ulceration are significant neuropathy with loss of protective sensations and ischemia. They can be referred to as primary risk factors and other risk factors like deformities, callus etc, as secondary risk factors. Secondary risk factors do not usually cause foot ulcerations unless associated with primary risk factors.

Primary Risk Factors

- Significant polyneuropathy with loss of protective sensations
- Evidence of ischemia in foot (ABI < 0.9)

Secondary Risk Factors

- Foot deformities
- Callus
- Previous ulcer
- Previous amputation
- Chronic renal failure
- Inappropriate footwear
- Impaired vision
- Person living alone
- Low educational status
- Noncompliant patient.

RISK CATEGORIZATION

The experts involved in developing the Consensus of the Diabetic Foot, currently suggest the following risk categorization system.

Table 41.1: Risk categorization system		
Category	*Risk profile*	*Check up frequency*
0	No sensory neuropathy	Once a year
1	Sensory neuropathy	Once every 6 months
2	Sensory neuropathy and signs of peripheral vascular disease and/or foot deformities	Once every 3 months
3	Previous ulcer/ amputation	Once every 1-3 months

Surveillence Category 0

It includes all patients diagnosed to have diabetes but have intact sensations of the foot. For early detection of neuropathy and ischemia, yearly evaluation of sensory system and vascular supply should be carried out.

Category 1

The patients in this category have lost protective sensations of the foot, thus putting them at a higher risk of injury. They need to be educated about proper footcare and advised preventive footwear.

Category 2

The patients in this category also have deformity in their foot along with loss of protective sensations. The skin is still intact. Presence of deformity increases plantar pressure considerably. The repetitive stress of walking alone can result in damage to their foot. They should be advised preventive footwear and should be told to reduce their activity level. Those patients who have evidence of PVD need to take extra precautions to avoid any foot inury. They should be evaluated for extent and severity of vascular disease and should be prescribed appropriate medical therapy.

Category 3

The patients in this category have a history of previous ulcer or even partial foot amputation. Scar of previous ulcer and amputation increase plantar pressure in other areas of the foot. The recurrence rate of an ulcer is very high in such patients and is to the tune of 50% in three years.

Scarring makes tissues less flexible and more likely to breakdown, particularly as a result of shear. These patients need to wear protective footwear. Those who have undergone partial foot amputation often need custom made special footwear. The activity level should be as minimum as possible, they should be told to use their feet sparingly.

As the risk of ulceration rises, so does the need for more frequent foot examination. Also, as the risk increases, the patient needs ever increasing levels of education. Despite careful patient education and frequent foot examination, careless action on the part of the patient often results in a foot injury, which can be very frustrating for the diabetic footcare team. However, the footcare team needs to realize that, it is part of the game and they should restrain from acusing the patient.

The patients categorized as high risk should be attended regularly by a footcare specialist. When patients are unable to cut their own nails safely, they should be trimmed regularly by the podiatrist, besides treating callus and nail lesions. Similarly footwear and insoles should be examined, wornout insoles need to be replaced.

The longterm surveillance is essential to protect a high risk foot from ulceration. The patients need to realize that, the high risk feet need to be used sparingly (Fig. 41.1). The activity level should be as minimum as possible.

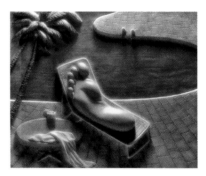

Fig. 41.1: Even feet need rest

42 Preventive Footwear

Out of shape footwear means an out of shape foot. If footwear is loose, it has little use

Footwear were created with the intention to protect feet from injury. However, over the years, shoes became a tool of the fashion world and fancy shoes became more and more popular. Aesthetic aspect of footwear gained more importance over the protective aspect. Such footwear became the cause of many foot problems like deformities, metatarsalgia, etc., even in the normal feet. Majority of the persons with diabetes mellitus do not need special footwear. However they should wear comfortable footwear like sports shoes, formal leather shoes or sandals.

Preventive footwear are however essential for patients with loss of protective sensations. The approach to footwear prescription should be graded.

OBJECTIVES OF PREVENTIVE FOOTWEAR

- Even distribution of plantar pressure and relief of areas of excessive plantar pressure
- Shock absorption
- Reduction in friction and shear
- Limiting joint motion
- Accomodation of deformities.

COMMONLY USED NOMENCLATURE (FIG. 42.1)

Last : The mold over which a shoe is made. Shoes for high risk feet require special lasts and must not be made over the standard lasts used for normal footwear. The last is dependent on the shape of a shoe, uppers and shape of the sole.

Outsole : Is the outer protective cover on the under-surface of the shoe.

Counter : Part of the shoe extending around the heel.

Uppers : Shoe part that covers the foot from above.

Toe box : Part that covers the toe area.

Throat : Part at the bottom of the laces.

Insole : Forms the floor of a shoe.

CHARACTERISTICS OF PREVENTIVE FOOTWEAR

The footwear should be light (weight upto 700g/pair), nontraumatic, and aesthetically acceptable to patients.

Outsole

Shoes with a soft outsole bend easily (Fig. 42.2) and are not able to stabilize the foot while walking. Rigid soles absorb shock and reduce vertical pressure. The outsole should be tough to prevent penetrating injuries from sharp objects. It should be serrated as smooth outsoles are slippery. The heel should not be higher than 2 inches (5 cm.). High heels increase the pressure over forefoot.

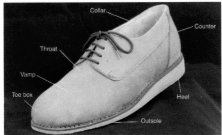

Fig. 42.1: Preventive footwear with commonly used nomenclature

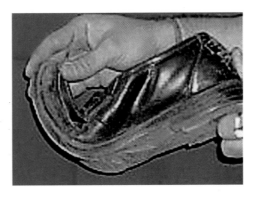

Fig. 42.2: Soft outsole which bends easily

Shoe Size

It is extremely important to have a proper sized shoe (Figs 42.3, 42.4). Patients with insensate feet tend to wear tight shoes as they do not get any discomfort. In loose shoes the foot slides increasing the shear stress. Length of a shoe should allow ½ inch (1.25 cm.) between the end of the shoe and the longest toe and can be measured using an appropriate device (Fig. 42.5). The foot is widest at the first metatarsophalangeal joint and should match with the widest part of the shoe. Shoe size mentioned on the shoe varies among brands and styles.

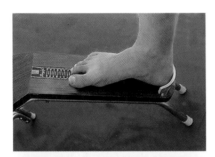

Fig. 42.3: Measuring scale for shoe size

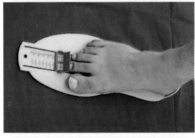

Fig. 42.4: Measuring scale for shoe size

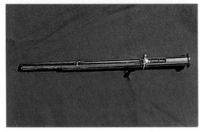

Fig. 42.5: Measuring scale with spring to know the internal length of the shoe

Counter

The counter controls the heel and determines its fit inside the shoe.

Shoes with Laces or Velcro

Shoes should be fastened with laces or velcro, to allow adjustability needed for edema or deformities and allow the shoe to be fit properly without the danger of it slipping off. Slip-on shoes may better be avoided.

Depth of the Shoe

Footwear should have an extra depth to accommodate dorsal deformities and removable insoles.

Toe box

A rounded and high toe box (Fig. 42.6) is essential to accommodate dorsal deformities (clawed toes, hammer toes). A shoe with a narrow or tapered toe box aggravates friction and deformities like hallux valgus and a rigid toe cap (Fig. 42.7) causes toe compression.

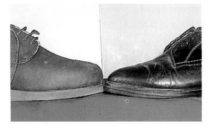

Fig. 42.6: Shoe with high toe box compared with a conventional shoe

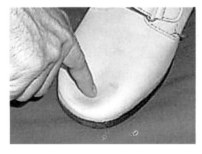

Fig. 42.7: Shoe without a rigid toe cap

Uppers

The uppers should have a soft inner lining to prevent friction injuries, like bunions. Uppers can also be made of elastic or a soft and flexible material instead of leather (Fig. 42.16).

Insoles

Insoles give cushioning to the feet and allow distribution of plantar pressure; they also act like a shock absorber (Fig. 42.8). They should be inserted

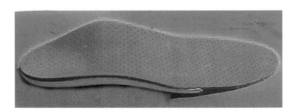

Fig. 42.8: Insole for shock absorption

inside the shoe without making the shoe too tight. They are made of microcellular rubber, ethyl-vinyl-acetate or polyethelene foam (Plastazote). Insoles wear out (bottoming out) and therefore need to be replaced periodically (3 to 6 months).

Socks

Soft cotton socks reduce the shear stress (Fig. 42.9). Soft padded socks are also useful in reducing the plantar pressure. Seamless socks may be preferred over seamed ones.

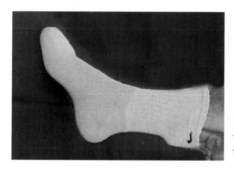

Fig. 42.9: Soft cotton socks without tight elastic

RECOMMENDATIONS FOR VARIOUS RISK CATEGORIES

Risk category 0

Majority of the diabetic patients fall in this category. They have no history of foot problems and have no neuropathy. They should wear shoes available over the counter. For brisk walking they should wear sports shoes (Fig. 42.10).

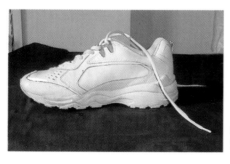

Fig. 42.10: Sport shoe for brisk walking

Risk Category 1

The patients in this category have loss of protective sensations without any deformities. They should wear soft cushioned sports shoes or preventive footwear (Fig. 42.1, 42.11 to 42.13). Certain footwear like Hawaii

slippers, stilettos and those with a narrow toe box should best be avoided (Fig. 42.14 A, 42.15 E). Hawaii slippers are convenient to wear and are therefore extremely popular. They have one grip pattern between the great toe and the second toe. Diabetic patients with neuropathy find it hard to walk with them as they slip off without their knowledge. To keep them in position, patients have to walk with an extra firm grip, producing pressure areas on the tips of the toes. High heeled footwear and stilettos increase pressure on the forefoot significantly, while footwear with a narrow toe box cause deformities like hallux valgus and crowding of toes.

Preventive Footwear

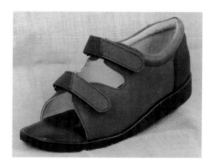

Fig. 42.11: Preventive footwear (Sandal) with velcro belts

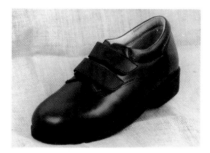

Fig. 42.12: Preventive shoe with velcro belts

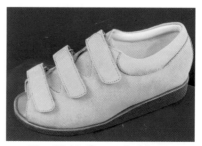

Fig. 42.13: Preventive footwear (Sandal) with velcro belts

Types of footwear to be avoided

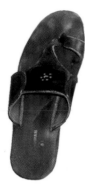
Fig. 42.14A:

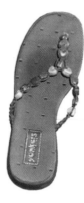
Fig. 42.14B:

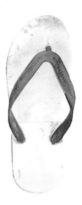
Fig. 42.14C:

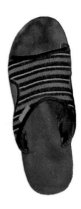
Fig. 42.14D:

(Chappals with grip pattern in 1st webspace A, B, C & D with dorsal belts, all without a counter)

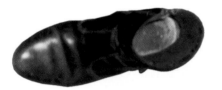

Fig. 42.15A: Narrow toe box

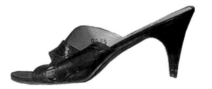
Fig. 42.15B: Stiletto

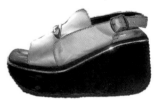
Fig. 42.15C: Platform heels

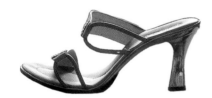
Fig. 42.15D: High heels

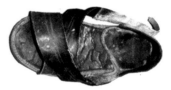
Fig. 42.15E: wornout footwear

Risk Category 2

These patients have loss of protective sensations and deformities and should be advised shoes with elastic uppers (Fig. 42.16) or shoes with an extra depth, high toe box and soft insoles (Fig. 42.1, 42.11 to 42.13).

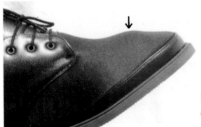
Fig. 42.16: Shoe with elastic uppers to acco-modate toe deformities

Risk Category 3

These patients have a history of previous ulcer or partial foot amputation. They should be advised preventive footwear as in category 2, if the shape of the foot is not grossly altered. Those with a grossly abnormal shape of the foot need custom molded shoes and insoles. Such shoes are manufactured over individualized lasts (Fig. 42.17) made from plaster

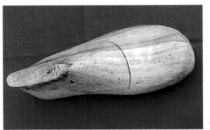
Fig. 42.17A: Last for a custom made shoe

models of each foot. Molded insoles are designed to redistribute pressure and provide cushioning. A plaster of paris cast of the foot is taken to represent its overall contours. Then a last is made over which insoles are molded. The patients with history of forefoot ulceration, can be given forefoot relief shoes (Fig. 42.18, 42.19) and those with partial foot amputations, such as lisfranc and Chopart, may be given special shoes (Fig. 42.20). These shoes should have an ankle support and a filler for the portion of the foot that has been amputated.

The patients with toe, ray or transmetatarsal amputations usually do not need special shoes and may be advised shoes with an extra depth, high toe box and soft insoles. Toe spacers may be advised, to prevent hallux valgus, to patients who have undergone a 2nd toe amputation, while distal fillers to those with transmetatarsal amputation.

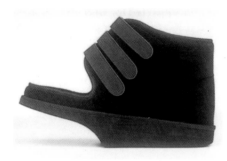

Fig. 42.18: Forefoot relief shoe
(Reproduced by kind permission of the "International working group on the diabetic foot")

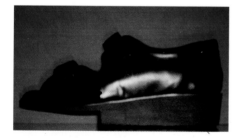

Fig. 42.19: Forefoot relief sandal

INSTRUCTIONS FOR PATIENTS

- Footwear sizes are not standard, look in a size range, based on results of measuring.
- New footwear should not be worn for longer time (2 hrs), allow the leather to soften.

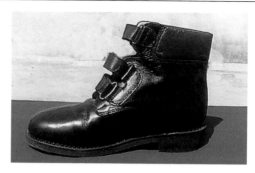

Fig. 42.20: Special shoe for patients with Lisfranc and Chopart amputation

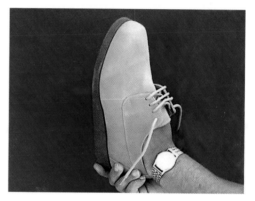

Fig. 42.21: Patient should feel inside the shoe

- Buy footwear preferably in the evening because feet swell a little in the evening.
- Stockings or socks should always be worn with shoes, to avoid blisters.
- Footwear for the high risk feet is intended to prevent and not heal foot lesions.
- Footwear in which the foot has ulcerated needs to be replaced.
- Care of feet is mandatory, even if one is using a preventive footwear.
- Footwear is effective, if it is preventing buildup of callus.
- Footwear and insoles should be periodically checked by the experts of footcare team.
- Check shoes before putting them on, to look for any foreign objects (Fig. 42.21).
- Examine shoes, feel inside the shoes for torn, loose linings or foreign objects and outsoles for embedded foreign objects (nails), cracks and wearing out.
- Patients should examine their feet, after removing the shoes, for reddened areas which may indicate an increased pressure.

43 Diabetic Foot Clinic and Team Approach

Team work makes everything possible even the impossible

It has to be realized by all those involved in footcare for persons with diabetes that no one specialist possesses all the skills needed to prevent leg amputation. Therefore the team approach is of paramount importance. Unfortunately, in majority of the centres, the scenario is just the opposite. The diabetic foot services are compartmental and fragmented, with hardly any coordination and communication among various specialists. The patients are seen at different times and venues by different specialists. The net effect is no effect. No one shoulders the primary responsibility, no joint decisions are made, the anesthetists and the surgeons tend to postpone the surgery, for the lack of smooth glycemic control prior to surgery, the ward nurses avoid the stinking patients and push them to distant corners of the ward and the poor diabetes specialist finds it difficult to achieve the desired glycemic control in presence of infection. Days and weeks are often lost before the definitive surgery is carried out, by then more soft tissues are necrosed and the infection progresses more proximally.

The diabetic footcare team should work in the diabetic foot clinic to provide an integrated approach to the management of varied clinical presentations of the diabetic foot. There is an urgent need to develop such multidisciplinary diabetic foot clinics, where the team members are willing to work with great interest and dedication. The well organized diabetic foot clinic, providing consistent patient education as well as preventive and acute care for diabetic foot lesions can be expected to bring gratifying results both in preventing the foot lesions as well as healing them. More limbs will be salvaged and the quality of life of diabetic patients with foot problems will improve enormously.

Members of Diabetic Foot-Care Team

- **Diabetologist (captain)**
- Surgeon
- Podiatrist
- Educator
- Nurse
- Orthotist
- Social worker
- Relative of the patient

The motto of this team should be to save the limb and not amputate it. Other specialists are needed for evaluation and management of specific problems and should be available at a short notice to provide their expertise.

Extended Team Members

- Internist
- Cardiologist
- Nephrologist
- Neurologist
- Microbiologist
- Physiotherapist
- Biochemist
- Plastic surgeon
- Orthopedic surgeon
- Vascular surgeon
- Radiologist
- Interventional radiologist
- Occupational therapist
- Dermatologist

For proper examination of the feet and diagnosis of the foot problem, certain equipments are necessary.

Basic diagnostic equipments (Fig. 43.1)

- 10 gm monofilament
- 128 hz tuning fork
- Hand-held Doppler
- Biothesiometer
- Ink pad for foot prints
- Sphygmomanometer
- Glucometer

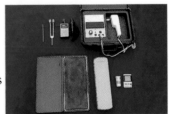

Fig. 43.1: Basic diagnostic equipments

To carry out the outdoor procedures like callus removal, deroofing of the bullae, debridement of superficial infections, nail clipping, and wound dressings, certain instruments are required.

Set of Instruments and accessories (Fig. 43.2)

- Sterile gloves`
- Nail clipper
- Nail file
- Scalpel with handle
- Surgical scissors
- Mayo's scissors
- Artery forceps
- Metal probe
- Scoop
- Tooth forceps
- Magnifying glass
- Magnifying Mirror

Footwear examination and prescribing preventive footwear is an integral part of the diabetic foot clinic.

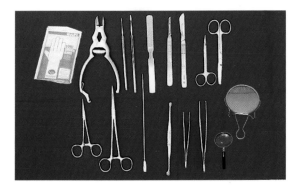

Fig. 43.2: Set of Instruments and accessories

Footwear and Off-loading Related Equipments

- Printed sheets to document the foot size
- Insole materials
- Walker
- Foot size measuring scale
- Felt pads and foams
- Temporary shoes
- Weight relief shoes
- Crutches
- Footwear measuring instrument
- Measuring Tape
- Adhesive solutions
- Casting material for molded soles

Patient education (discussed in chapter 44), record keeping and documentation are other aspects which are equally important.

Audiovisual Aids and Data Collections

- Television set (Transparencies)
- Video Compact Disc (VCD)
- Digital camera
- Computer
- Overhead projector
- Slide projector
- Writing board
- Printed educational material, boards, flip charts.

The fight against diabetic foot is long drawn, difficult, frustrating but challenging too. It can be won if the team members are spirited and work in close liason with other members of extended group, primary care physicians and referral centres. The need is to keep comprehensive records of the patients, keep close follow up with them and conduct audits of the clinic cases for evaluation of results with critical analysis.

44 Patient Education

"Of all the approaches to saving the diabetic foot, the most important is patient education"
— Marvin Levin

The education of a patient, his family members and primary care physicians is extremely important to reduce the risk factors for lower limb morbidity and prevent limb amputation. Every time I see a new patient with an advanced diabetic foot, I feel, "it should not have progressed to such an extent" but over and again the same basic mistakes are made by the patient and or the treating physician.

The recurrence of foot ulceration, despite careful patient education, is frustrating both for the treating physician and the patient. It is also commonly observed that the patient is blamed either for the recurrence or late reporting. One has to realize that neglect of the foot is not intentional but is caused by absent sensory input that makes him or her unaware of the lesion. This would be a problem for any of us because we are attuned only to things we can be aware of and we are only aware of things we sense. It is unjust to label the patient as noncompliant and uncooperative, when in reality, the patient has not been adequately taught how to overcome the absent sensation in the feet.

PRINCIPLES OF EDUCATION

- Education is essential at every visit, for evaluation of the feet.
- The opportunity should be utilized by all the members of the footcare team. All of them should speak the same language and their statements should not be contradictory.
- The information should comply with the patient's need and the risk category.
- Incorrect information feed can overwhelm or even scare a patient. Footcare education needs to match the risk curve continually.
- If a specific practice or routine is required of the patient, it is best to have it rehearsed under supervision of the clinical staff.

WHOM TO EDUCATE

- *Individual patient:* Patients of different risk categories should be educated accordingly. Education goals should be set and at subsequent visits patients should be evaluated to know if the goals have been met.
- *Group education:* Patients with previous foot ulcers, previous amputation, those with present foot ulcers and high risk feet may be collectively educated by members of the footcare team. Such stimulus sessions should provoke responses and encourage thinking. The patients should be encouraged to narrate their experiences like how they developed the foot ulcer and how it healed. This kind of patient participation is very effective. (Fig. 44.1). Group education has recognized advantages over individual teaching because of the

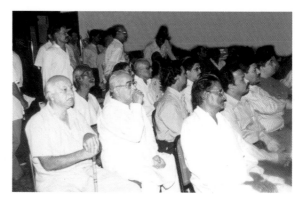

Fig. 44.1: Group of patients with foot problems, being educated

enhancing effect patient interaction has on the learning process. Video tapes can be shown and patient's queries dealt with, by the well trained staff of the footcare team.

The patients pass through different stages of motivation; barriers to motivation and behavioral change must be addressed. The more the patients have to work with the information provided during the programme, more likely is it that the information will result in a behavioral change. It has to be ensured that patients understand

- What has happened
- Why has it happened
- What to do about it
- How to prevent it from happening again.
- **Education of the primary care physicians :** Primary care physician is the first doctor of contact and he sees trivial lesions of the foot when they have first begun. These physicians need to be trained properly to recognize the feet at risk, trivial lesions and progressive lesions. They can be empowered to take the prompt decision of an early referral to the diabetic footcare team, starting antibiotics if needed, and to follow-up the patients for periodic dressings of the wound. We conduct clinical meetings of these physicians and discuss few cases of the diabetic foot in a simple manner (Figs 44.2 to 44.5). They are encouraged to ask questions and get their queries solved by experts.

EDUCATIONAL AIDS

Various visual aids like posters, pictures, overhead transparencies, power point presentations and

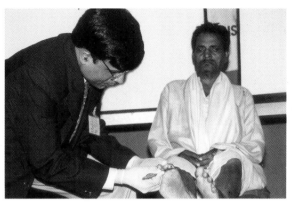
Fig. 44.3: Group of doctors receiving demonstration of callus removal

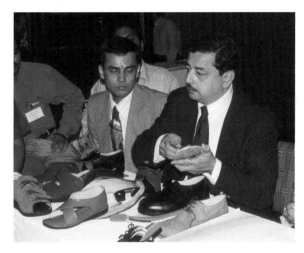
Fig. 44.4: Group of doctors being explained about preventive footwear

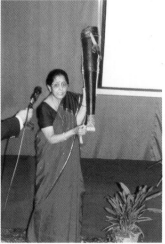
Fig. 44.5: Group of doctors being explained about prosthesis

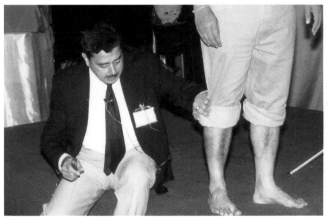
Fig. 44.2: Group of doctors being explained the biomechanics

videotapes can be used to enhance the information explained verbally. Printed leaflets and booklets can be distributed as a ready reckoner. Audiovisual aids should not be used to escape talking to the patient. They should not be a substitute for interaction with the learner.

FOOT-CARE INSTRUCTIONS

• Daily inspection of the feet, including areas between toes (Fig. 44.6)
• Daily washing of feet and drying, especially between toes (Fig. 44.7)

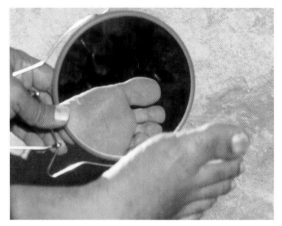

Fig. 44.6: Inspection of feet in a mirror

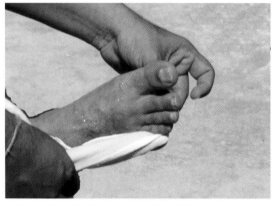

Fig. 44.7: Washing and drying of feet, especially between toes

• Hot water should not be used for washing the feet
• Lubricating oils or moisturising creams should be used for dry skin, avoiding their application in between the toes
• Daily inspection and palpation of the insides of shoes
• Daily change of stocking or socks
• Avoid barefoot walking in and out doors
• Nails should be cut straight across
• Avoid home surgery, for corns or callus
• Patients with neuropathic feet should limit or avoid repetitive weight bearing exercises such as jogging and prolonged walking.
• Avoid visiting temples or sandy beaches during the day time, when the surfaces are hot; visit either early, in the morning or late in the evening.
• Regular visit to the footcare team
• Report at once if a blister, cut or ulceration has developed.

The patients with high risk feet should be encouraged to take shorter, slower steps and avoid excessive walking to decrease chronic foot trauma which can lead to tissue breakdown. The style of instructions, including the terminology used is tailored to the patients' ability to understand the foot problem. It is also very important that the instructions given by all the team members be consistent and repeated as often as necessary to ensure comprehension. Attitudes and beliefs are the two most important determinants of behaviour and need to be effectively addressed. Patients will not be committed unless they are convinced that :

• They have foot problem
• Its consequences are serious
• It can be treated effectively
• The advantages of treatment outweigh the disadvantages.

Patient education is the master key to foot ulcer prevention. More importantly there is the necessity to maintain the desire not only to put knowledge and skills into practice, but to continue doing so through the years to come. If patients come to bestow as much love on their feet as their face, much of the battle could be won.

Section Eight

Other Aspects

- Learning from Failures

- Maggots (Larval Therapy)

- Newer Dressings

- Newer Therapies

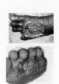

45 Learning from Failures

Behind every success there is failure

The truth is that medical science, though evidence based and backed by extensive scientific research, is yet plagued with far too many uncertainties. No wonder, it is doctors who treat patients and this cannot be left to the rigid stereotype of the text books or the straight-jacket of a computer. And rightly so, similarly, diseases, by not adhering to the defined pattern, often do not obey the text books. Many a clinical decision is forced on the spur of the moment, at times even banking on intuition born out of experience. At every turn, expect the unexpected would seem to be the norm. Therefore, in this quest for success, the inescapable failures are as if drilled into the game plan.

Diabetic foot is one such tricky situation, where absence of symptoms, often compounds the complexity. There are no ways to decide the anatomical extent precisely and hence majority of the surgical debridements are based on the surgeon's experience and preoperative and intraoperative clinical judgement. The clinical course of the diabetic foot can often be unpredictable, catching everyone off-guard. Unfortunately, despite all our efforts, some wounds still fail to heal due to factors as yet unknown to us. Sadly, in the foreseeable future, failures are here to stay. But each teaches a distinct lesson, opening up a virgin progress pathway. Some of our failures are discussed below.

Case Study (45.A)

This 68 year old male with type 2 DM of 6 years presented with swollen left foot, secondary to an unknown injury of 1 week duration. On examination he was clinically stable, BP 160/100 mmHg, systemic examination was normal, ECG showed T wave inversion in V_1 to V_6 leads. The patient denied any history of chest pain in the past.

Local examination of left foot revealed a purulent bulla over the dorsum with 4th web space (Fig. 45.1 A) infection. The plantar aspect was apparently normal. He had a neuropathic feet with normal ABI. The patient was hospitalized, was switched on to intravenous antibiotics and multiple injections of insulin.

Deroofing of the bulla was carried out which revealed an area of necrosis with deep infection (Fig. 45.1 B). The X-ray foot did not reveal osteomyelitis. Hence he was subjected for surgical debridement but even after debridement the wound continued to discharge pus and showed areas of necrosis (Fig. 45.1 C). Microbial culture showed growth of *Pseudomonas*

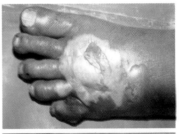

Fig. 45.1A: Purulent bulla over left dorsum

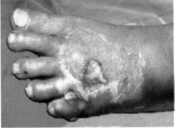

Fig. 45.1B: After deroofing, note area of necrosis

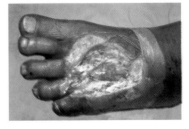

Fig. 45.1C: After surgical debridement

aeroginosa, hence appropriate changes in the i/v antibiotics were made. A decision of partial 4th ray amputation was taken and implemented alongwith debridement of necrotic tissue. The wound showed a remarkable improvement, was red and devoid of necrotic tissue (Fig. 45.2A). At this stage three weeks after admission, the patient insisted for a discharge.

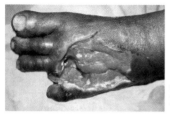

Fig. 45.2A: After 4th ray amputation, apparently healthy wound

He was managed at home under cover of oral antibiotics and insulin injections alongwith daily wound dressings. He returned 15 days later, the wound showed multiple maggots, which were removed (Fig. 45.2B). The wound revealed an area of necrosis at the amputation site (Fig. 45.2C), probing of the wound showed evidence of osteomyelitis. The plantar aspect revealed swelling in the forefoot and the X-ray showed destruction of 3rd MTP joint and early osteolytic changes in 2nd MTH (Fig. 45.2D). At

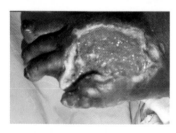

Fig. 45.2B: Maggots seen over the wound, note sinus near the base of 3rd toe

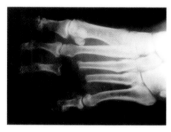

Fig. 45.2C: Necrotic tissue at amputation site

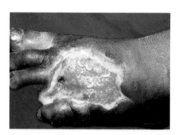

Fig. 45.2D: Radiograph showing partial 4th ray amputation, osteolytic destruction of 3rd MTP joint and early osteolytic changes in 2nd MT head

this stage a duplex Doppler was done, which was normal. In view of these clinical findings and evidence of advancing infection, a decision to carry out more proximal amputation was taken. A tarsometatarsal amputation was carried out (Fig. 45.3A) and the wound was closed with loose sutures. Bacterial swab at this stage surprisingly showed no growth. The wound once again started discharging purulent material and hence the stitches were opened. The stump showed multiple areas of necrosis (Fig. 45.3B).

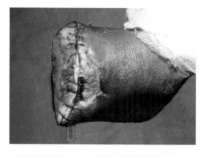

Fig. 45.3A: After tarso-metatarsal amputation (Lisfranc), wound closed by loose sutures, note the corrugated rubber drain

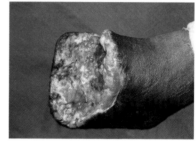

Fig. 45.3B: After removal of stiches, areas of necrosis seen

Considering the age of the patient and non responding infective process, a decision to carry out BK amputation was made and implemented. The patient made an uneventful recovery and was discharged 2 weeks later. He was rehabilitated with limb prosthesis. He lived for 4 more years and died of myocardial infarction. The lessons we learnt were:

- Purulent blister indicates deep soft tissue infection and hence only deroofing such a bulla is not the solution.
- Thinking back makes us feel that, probably along with 4th ray amputation, disarticulation of 5th toe should have been carried out.
- Continued worsening of the wound despite tarsometatarsal amputation indicates the possibility of resistant and virulent strain of microorganisms.

This patient who presented with a dorsal foot infection of 7 days duration, underwent 4 surgeries over a period of 2 months, thus reinforcing the fact that some wounds fail to heel due to factors unknown to us, as yet.

Case Study (45.B)

This 40 year old female type 1 diabetic since 10 years was a regular visitor to our centre. She was a non compliant patient who used to miss insulin injections frequently and get admitted for ketoacidosis. In 10 years time, she had already developed Charcot foot (left) with multiple ulcers over the heel and a neuropathic ulcer on her right great toe (Fig. 45.4). She was not particular about care of her feet and the low socioeconomic background compelled her to carry out household activities like cooking, washing clothes and utensils manually and look after 4 growing children and her husband. She was twice treated at our centre for foot ulcerations, one of them after a snake bite.

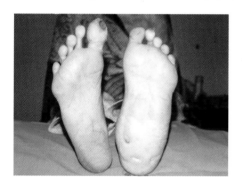

Fig. 45.4: Charcot foot left with multiple sinuses on the heel, plantar ulcer great toe right (Picture taken 1 year before present admission)

Two months prior to present admission, she had visited her native village in north India, where she developed a non healing wound on her right foot 4th toe while working on the farm. The wound was neglected and it started draining pus. She continued to work and the wound deteriorated further. She noticed another swelling over the heel with discharging ulcers and then she decided to return home, and reported at our centre. She was immediately hospitalized.

On admission she was toxic, pale, febrile, hypotensive with systolic BP 90 mmHg and dyspnoeic. The right foot wound was terribly smelly, with an infected and necrotic ulcer in the 4th webspace and multiple discharging ulcers over the heel, without crepitus (Figs 45.5A to C). She had neuropathic feet

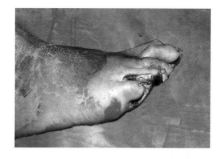

Fig. 45.5A: 4th web-space infection, destruction 3rd, 4th toes and cellulitis

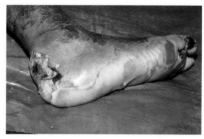

Fig. 45.5B: Lateral compartment infection spread into heel pad with extensive necrosis

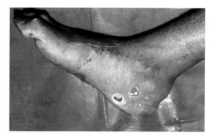

Fig. 45.5C: Medial view, multiple sinuses, deep heel pad infection, note the leg appears apparently normal

with normal ABI. The left foot was surprisingly quiet, although showed evidence of Charcot foot. She was rushed to critical care unit, was managed with insulin infusion for ketoacidosis, was rehydrated and was given dopamine drip. She was switched on to broad spectrum antibiotics in higher doses and was given 2 units blood transfusion. Clinical diagnosis of badly infected foot, ketoacidosis, septicemic shock was made. Her laboratory investigations revealed Hb of 4 gms% , ESR 170 mm / 1st hr TLC 12,600/cu.mm, creatinine 2.6 mg%, S. Na$^+$ 126 mEq/Lit, S.K$^+$ 4.8 mEq/Lit, ALT 85 IU/L, AST 80 IU/L. Her ECG was normal except for sinus tachycardia. A bacterial culture showed growth of *Pseudomonas aeroginosa*. After stabilization of her clinical condition, she was taken for below knee amputation and the stump was closed by primary sutures. The patient tolerated the procedure very well and showed signs of recovery. She started sitting up in the bed, her appetite improved and she was weaned off intravenous fluids, although the intravenous antibiotics continued. On 7th post operative day, she started getting fever and the stump got swollen. She was then posted for exploration of the stump, stitches were removed (Fig. 45.6) and the necrotic tissue debrided. A bacterial culture this time showed growth of *staphylococci auerus*, hence appropriate changes in the i/v antibiotics were made. On daily dressings, pus could be milked out; once again patient's general condition started sinking. During clinical rounds, a possibility of carrying out above knee amputation was discussed. However, ultimately it was decided to continue the conservative line of treatment. The patient requested for discharge against medical advise and went home in moribund state and died after 4 days, 6 weeks after the admission.

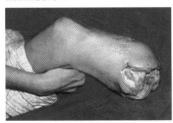

Fig. 45.6: Stump opened to remove pus and necrotic tissue

This death was probably a preventable one. Retrospectively it was thought that the magnitude of advancing leg infection could not be properly assessed preoperatively. Whether primary above knee amputation should have been the surgery of choice, is a debatable question. However, we do believe that the decision to go ahead with AK amputation should have been taken after exploration of the BK stump wound.

The amputated limb which was preserved in formalin was examined. It revealed pus tract extending from the lateral compartment to heel and into the leg (Figs 45.7A to C). The heel showed extensive necrosis of the tissues and tendoachilles. The autopsy study of the amputatated limb clearly showed that the infection had progressed much proximally into the leg than was anticipated at 1st surgery (BK amputation).

Autopsy Picture

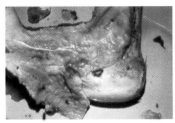

Fig. 45.7A: Showing pus tract extending into deep plantar compartments

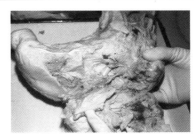

Fig. 45.7B: Showing extensive destruction of the heel pad

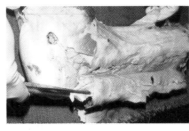

Fig. 45.7C: Showing necrosis of tendo-achillis and proximal extension into the leg

Case Study (45.C)

This 62 year old female, a retired nurse with type 2 DM of 18 years duration, presented with severe rest pain left lower limb and gangrene of lateral 4 toes (Fig. 45.8A). Her general physical and systemic examination were normal. She had non palpable dorsalis pedis and posterior tibials on both sides. She was hospitalized and investigated. The positive laboratory findings were, resting ECG showed T wave inversion in all the chest leads, although she had denied history of any chest pain. Duplex color doppler was not being done 16 years ago, however, conventional transfemoral angiography was carried out. It revealed generalised atherosclerotic changes and multiple stenotic lesions in the superficial femoral artery on left (Fig. 45.8B). She was treated with multiple injections of insulin,

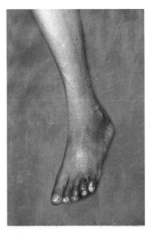

Fig. 45.8A: Showing gangrene of 4 lateral toes

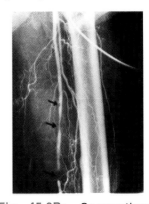

Fig. 45.8B: Conventional angiogram showing multiple occlusions in superficial femoral artery, a complete block in its lower part and reformation of popliteal through collaterals

intravenous broad spectrum antibiotics, analgesics and opiates. However her rest pain continued and worsened over the days. A vascular surgeon was consulted, who advised femoro-femoral bypass using a prosthetic graft and the bypass surgery was carried out. Unfortunately, her rest pain continued to worsen. The surgeon this time advised a BK amputation, which was carried out but in vain, as the stump got necrotic and malodorous.

The entire treating footcare team was frustrated, so also the patient. Finally above knee amputation was carried out to end terrible sufferings of the patient and the wound healed primarily (Fig. 45.8C). The patient's rest pain disappeared although she had phantom limb for 6 months. On discharge from the hospital, after 2 months long stay, she commented to me, "Doctor you made a mess of my leg". I was at loss of words, I just patted on her shoulder and said "goodbye". The lady lived for 4 years, with a compromised quality of life, and died of myocardial infarction.

Advanced PVD, with critical leg ischemia is a difficult clinical situation. In this patient unfortunately, two major surgeries had failed. Retrospectively, I feel whether a primary AK amputation alone should have been the surgery of choice?

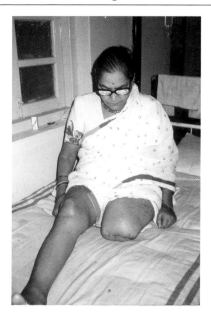

Fig. 45.8 C: Ultimately a AK amputation performed to stop her terrible sufferings

46 Maggots (Larval Therapy)

Crawly little creatures, come useful too!

Maggot is the larval form in the life cycle of a housefly. Maggots are commonly seen in infected wounds which are left uncovered. Open wounds attract flies, who lay eggs in such an environment. Maggots start sprawling in the wounds once the eggs are hatched. These larvae immediately begin to feed using a combination of mouth hooks and proteolytic secretions and excretions. If the conditions are favourable, the larvae grow rapidly, several times their original size. The full grown larvae stop feeding and search for a dry place to pupate and complete the life cycle with the emergence of a new adult fly.

Maggots selectively remove dead tissue, leaving healthy tissue intact. This is done by means of complex mechanisms which involve production of powerful proteolytic enzymes that breakdown dead tissue to a semi-liquid form, which in then ingested by the larvae. It is believed that proteolytic enzymes produced by larvae are inactivated by enzyme inhibitors present in healthy tissue which are not present in necrotic tissue. That is why larvae remove only necrotic tissue leaving healthy tissue intact.

Use of biological agents for treating wounds has been known for several centuries. Patients with infected wounds used to immerse their limb in the river to allow fish to eat away necrotic tissues, similarly leeches were used to reduce the swelling around the wound. Maggots were also known for their cleansing action in intractable osteomyelitis and traumatic injuries during war time. However, after the advent of antibiotics, use of maggots declined. Antibiotics offered a far better and aesthetically more acceptable form of treatment for serious wound infections.

The revival of interest in maggots therapy began some twenty years ago for treating pressure ulcers in patients with spinal cord injuries, in venous ulcers and fungating malignancies. They were also found to be useful in diabetic wound infections. In UK sterile larvae are available on prescription and are also exported to other European Countries.

It is not uncommon to see maggots pouring out from wounds in veterinary practice, leprosy patients and foul smelling wounds in patients with diabetes (Figs 46.1, 46.2A). I feel maggots are too slow for infected wounds in diabetes and certainly cannot be a substitute for good surgical debridement. At our centre, we in fact remove them with forceps and use medical turpentine to bring them out from the wound (Fig. 46.2B). Removal of maggots needs to be continued for at least three to four days as new eggs are hatched. It is not aesthetically acceptable for patients and the relatives to leave maggots in the wound.

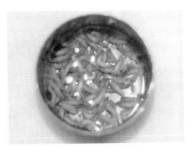

Fig. 46.1: Maggots delivered by forceps from the wound, they were alive and well

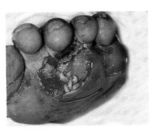

Fig. 46.2A: Maggots pouring out from the wound of a patient

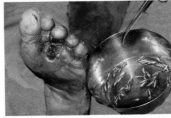

Fig. 46.2B: Maggots being removed from the wound

However, I have found maggots very useful in wounds of leprosy patients. Wounds in leprosy have more of necrotic tissue and slough than fulminant infection which is commonly seen in diabetes. Leprosy patients also do not have easy access to surgeons or podiatrists because of socio economic factors. Maggots are thus a boon for them.

There are presently ongoing randomized controlled trials to compare maggots with conventional treatments in the management of different types of necrotic wounds. These studies would throw more light on the therapeutic use of maggots in diabetic wounds in the near future.

The technical details in this chapter have been adopted from Stephen Thomas. New Treatments for Diabetic Foot Ulcers. In : Andrew JM Boulton, Henry Connor and Peter R Cavanagh eds. The Foot in Diabetes. Wiley & Sons : 2000; 185 - 191.

47 Newer Dressings

Still waters run deep

Conventional dressings, such as gauze, impregnated gauze, gauze and cotton, packing strips have been in use for over fifty years. Moist wound environment that these dressings provide are best for wound regeneration and repair and increasing the velocity of healing. Effective wound management aims to strike a balance, i.e. a moist environment to promote healing, but not so wet as to cause maceration and excoriation.

Two factors are important for natural wound healing. One is wound exudate which is the generic term given to the liquid produced from wounds. Exudate keeps the wound moist, supplies nutrients, and provides the medium for migration and mitosis of epethelial cells. This in turn, keeps the wound supplied with leucocytes, helping to control micro organisms. Second factor is the presence of white cells in the wound. White cells play a major role in wound healing by cleaning the wound, removing potentially pathogenic micro organisms and producing collagen, the building block of new tissue. Excessive exudates can cause maceration and hence the dressing should be able to absorb excessive exudates from the wound. The characteristics of an ideal dressing are given in Table 47.1.

Table 47.1: Characteristics of an ideal dressing
• To remove excess exudate and toxic components
• To maintain high humidity in the wound
• To allow gaseous exchange
• To provide thermal insulation
• To provide protection from secondary infection
• To allow removal without trauma at dressing change
• To be free from particulate and toxic components.

NEWER DRESSINGS

A wide variety of new dressing materials have been developed. However none of the newer dressings fulfill all the characteristics of an ideal dressing. Some of the newer dressings are discussed below in brief .

Film Dressing

These films are presented as thin sheets of clear material, bound on the wound-contact surface, with an adhesive. They are semi-permeable films with an ability to transmit moisture vapor from the wound to the external surface of the dressing. The advantages are, they form a bacterial barrier, are durable and often do not require changing more than every 4-5 days. The common indications for film dressings are superficial ulcers. They are not recommended for chronic diabetic wounds.

Foam Dressing

Polyurethane foam sheet dressings are being used in the management of moderate to heavy exudative wounds, while maintaining the viability of the surrounding skin. Foams provide thermal insulation to a wound and they can be cut and shaped to fit awkward areas. Their absorbing ability varies significantly with the type of foam used.

Nonadherent Dressing

Paraffin-impregnated tulle dressings are used to provide a non-adherent dressing. This type of dressing has no absorption properties, fluid from the wound can drain through the dressing and as they are non-adherent, there is no trauma on removal. However, in heavily exudating wounds, other dressings should be used.

Hydrogels

They are a mixture of polymers with up to 90% water content. They transmit moisture and oxygen and absorb fluid from the wound. Hydrogels promote wound debridement by rehydrating the wound bed and facilitating natural autolysis. Hydrogels are available in two forms, as sheet (stable structure) and amorphous (no fixed structure). Amorphous hydrogels are indicated for the debridement of non-viable tissue as an adjuvant to local sharp debridement.

Transorbent is a new multilayered hydrogel dressing. The adhesive layer becomes inactive when in contact with water, thus minimizing discomfort during dressing change. The hydrogel absorbs exudates and donates water, gaseous exchange allows oxygen to reach the wound and water vapour to environment. The dressing is highly absorbent, producing moist environment, with the anterfilm protecting against bacterial contamination.

Hydrocolloids

They form an airtight seal over the surface of the wound, reducing exudate production by up to 50%, however maceration of the surrounding skin can be a problem in cases of extremely high exudates. Hydocolloids work best if undisturbed for a few days. This however, prevents daily inspection of the wound and infection can go unrecognized if the wound dressing is not changed on a daily basis.

Alginates

Alginates are produced from the calcium and sodium salts of alginic acid. The capacity to absorb large amounts of exudates is one of the major advantages of alginates. The wound should always be observed closely as exudates decrease during the healing process, and alginates may not gel. If this occurs, the alginate will remain hard, forming a focus for pressure or blocking drainage of the remaining exudate. To avoid such consequences, alginates should not be allowed to dry out or be left in the wound for a long period. Alginate dressings are presented in many sizes and in both, sheet and ribbon or rope forms for use on flat or cavity wounds.

Alginates should be loosely packed into the cavity and left in place until all of the gel has become moist with exudate. Before removal, alginate dressing must first be irrigated with normal saline. However alginates being high in glucoronic acid, will not wash off with saline but can be removed intact with a gloved hand or forceps.

The treating foot-care team has to make appropriate choice of dressing for a particular type of wound. It is important to note that there is a wide range of performance parameters within and between various types of newer dressings. Although no dressing fulfills all the characteristics of an ideal dressing, important factors to consider include user friendliness, cost effectiveness and ability to maintain a moist wound environment.

48 Newer Therapies

Promising but cannot substitute fundamental of management

Wound healing is the process by which tissues respond to an injury. The process of wound healing is controlled by growth factors that initiate cell growth and proliferation by binding to specific high-affinity receptors on the cell surface. Growth factors have the ability to stimulate the mitosis of quiescent cells. They are produced by platelets, macrophages, epithelial cells, fibroblasts and endothelial cells. The growth factors most commonly involved in wound healing include platelet - derived growth factor (PDGF), fibroblast growth factor (FGF), epidermal growth factor (EGF) and insulin like growth factor (IGF).

Newer therapies provide various growth factors topically, to promote and hasten wound healing.

Platelet Derived Growth Factors (PDGF)

The process of wound repair is characterized by a series of complex cellular and molecular events. Growth factors play fundamental roles in this process, by stimulating chemotaxis and cellular proliferation. Several growth factors have been tried in chronic wounds including diabetic ulcers. The only topical growth factor that has shown convincing results to stimulate healing of chronic neuropathic diabetic ulcers is platelet derived growth factor (PDGF-BB becaplermin). It is recombinant human PDGF-BB gel preparation which is used for non infected neuropathic ulcers. The gel preparation is spread over the wound, and covered with a non-adherent saline soaked gauze dressing. The dressing is changed once or twice everyday. It has to be realized that this gel therapy is effective only if other modalities like recurrent surgical debridement of ulcer and offloading are adhered to. No significant side effects have been described. With PDGF therapy more ulcers heal, they heal faster and probably remain healed longer than the conventional therapy.

Dermagraft

It is bioengineered human dermis designed to replace a patient's own damaged or destroyed dermis. It consists of neonatal dermal fibroblasts cultured in vitro on a bioabsorbable polyglactin mesh. Fibroblasts are screened extensively for infectious agents before they are cultured. As the fibroblasts proliferate within the mesh, they secrete human dermal collagen, fibronectin, growth factors and other proteins, embedding themselves in a self produced dermal matrix. This results in a living, metabolically active dermal tissue with the structure of a papillary dermis of newborn skin. A single donor foreskin provides sufficient yield to produce 250,000 square feet of finished Dermagraft tissue.

Dermagraft is stored at -70°C. It is then shipped on dry ice to clinical sites. Prior to implantation, the product is rinsed with normal saline, cut to wound size and placed into the wound bed. The fibroblasts remain metabolically active and deliver a variety of growth factors which hasten wound healing. Thus, Dermagraft rebuilds healthy dermal base over which the patient's epidermis can migrate and close the wound. Dermagraft is applied usually once a week for 8 weeks, is very safe and has no side effects. It can be tried in indolent plantar neuropathic ulcers and even neuroischemic ulcers. The prerequiste is however that the ulcer should be free from infection. When Dermagraft is used, more ulcers are healed and healed significantly faster.

Apligraf

Like human skin, Apligraf consists of living skin cells and structural protein. The lower dermal combined bovine type 1 collagen and human fibroblasts (dermal cells), which produce additional matrix proteins. The upper epidermal layer is formed by prompting human keratinocytes (epidermal cells) first to multiply and then to differentiate to replicate the architecture of the human epidermis. Unlike human skin, Apligraf does not contain melanocytes, Langerhan's cells, macrophages, and lymphocytes, or other structures such as blood vessels, hair follicles or sweat glands. Studies have shown that with Apligraf neuropathic ulcers heal faster. Apligraf should not be used on infected ulcers.

Granulocyte – colony stimulating factor (GCSF)

It is an endogenous hemopoietic growth factor that induces terminal differentiation and release of neutrophils from the bone marrow. Endogenous concentrations of GCSF rise during bacterial sepsis, suggesting its role in the neutrophil response to infection. GCSF improves function in both normal and dysfunctional neutrophils. Since, diabetes represents an immunocompromised state secondary to neutrophil dysfunction, the effect of systemic recombinant human GCSF (filgrastim) has been tried in diabetic foot infections. It is administered as a daily subcutaneous injection for one week.

GCSF therapy has been shown to be associated with earlier eradication of pathogens from infected ulcers, quicker resolution of cellulitis, shorter hospital stay and shorter duration of intravenous antibiotic treatment. GCSF therapy was seen to be associated with leukocytosis, due almost entirely to an increase in neutrophil count. Thus GCSF may be an important adjunct to conventional therapy.

Hyaff

It is an ester of hyaluronic acid, which is a major component of the extracellular matrix. It facilitates growth and movement of fibroblasts and in contact with wound exudates, produces a hydrophilic gel which covers the wound and promotes granulation and healing. It has been found to be effective in neuropathic foot ulcers, especially with sinuses.

The newer therapies are promising, but fundamental principles of ulcer healing like off-loading cannot be ignored. The cost of therapy increases with use of newer modalities of treatment and its benefits like faster healing have to be weighed with the cost incurred for the treatment.

Although newer therapies have shown some promising results in promoting and hastening wound healing of non infected plantar neuropathic ulcers, they are no substitute to the fundamental principles of management of plantar ulcers like offloading, pressure relief and callus removal.

The technical details in this chapter have been partly adopted from
- *Michael E. Edmonds and Alethea VM Foster eds. Managing the Diabetic Foot. Blackwell Science : 2000; 123 – 125*
- *Michael E. Edmonds. New Treatments for Diabetic Foot ulcers. In : Andrew JM Boulton, Henry Connor and Peter R. Cavanagh eds. The Foot in Diabetes. Wiley & Sons : 2000; 179 – 184.*

Bibliography

Following books and special issues of journals have been generously referred while preparing the manuscript of this atlas.

1. Alistair McInnes (Ed). The Diabetic Foot 2001; 4 (2).
2. Alistair McInnes (Ed). The Diabetic Foot 1999; 2 (2).
3. Alistair McInnes (Ed). The Diabetic Foot 1999; 2 (4).
4. Alistair McInnes (Ed). The Diabetic Foot 1999;2(1).
5. Alistair McInnes (Ed). The Diabetic Foot 2000; 3 (3).
6. Clinical Ultrasound a Comprehensive Text, Abdominal and General Ultrasound. Colin Deane and David Goss. Limb arteries. Hylton Meire, David Cosgrove, Keith Dewbury, Pat Farrant (Eds). Churchill Livingstone: 2001; 1001-34.
7. Diagnostic Ultrasound. Joseph F. Polak. The Peripheral Arteries. Carol M Rumack, Stephanie R Wilson J, William Charboneau (Eds). Mosby-Year Book Inc: 1998;921-41.
8. Gray's Anatomy: Bannister LH, Berry MM, Collins P, Dyson M, Dussek JE, Ferguson MW J (Eds). Churchill Livingstone, 2000.
9. Insensitive Feet. A practical handbook on foot problems in Leprosy. Paul Brand. The Leprosy Mission, London, 1981.
10. International Consensus on the Diabetic Foot by the International Working Group on the diabetic foot, 1999.
11. Managing the Diabetic Foot. Michael E Edmonds, Alethea VM Foster (Eds). Blackwell Science, 2000.
12. Marvin E Levin, Lawrence W O'Neal's. The Diabetic Foot. John H Bowker, Michael A Pfeifer (Eds). Mosby-Year Book, 2001.
13. Morris D Kerstein (Ed). A symposium : Wound Infection and occlusion-separating Fact from Fiction. Am J of Surgery, 1994.
14. NC Schaper, K Bakker (Eds). The Diabetic Foot Proceedings of the Second International Symposium on the diabetic foot. Diabet Med 1996;13(suppl 1).
15. NC Schaper, K Bakker, J Rauwerda (Eds). The Diabetic Foot Proceedings of the Second International Symposium on the Diabetic Foot. Diabetes Metabolism Research and Reviews September-October 2000;16(Suppl 1).
16. Orthopaedics Principles and Their Application. Samuel L Turek (Ed). JB Foot and Ankle, Lippincott Company, 1978;1245-1321.
17. Sharad Pendsey (Ed). Foot Problems in Diabetes. Diabetes Bulletin: Int J Diab in Dev Count, 1994.
18. Sharad Pendsey. Peripheral Vascular Disease and the Diabetic Foot Syndrome. In MMS Ahuja, BB Tripathy, Sam GP Moses, HB Chandalia, AK Das, PV Rao and SV Madhu (Eds). Textbook of Diabetes Mellitus. RSSDI 2002; 42:559-70.
19. Surgery of the Foot and Ankle. Roger A Mann, Michael J Coughlin (Eds). Mosby-Year Book Inc, 1993.
20. The Foot in Diabetes. Andrew JM Boulton, Henry Connor, Peter R Cavangh (Eds). John Wiley & Sons, 2000.

Abbreviations

3 D	-	Three Dimensional	KPa	-	Kilo Pascals
ABI	-	Ankle/Brachial Pressure Index	LEA	-	Lower Extremity Amputation
AK	-	Above Knee	LJM	-	Limited Joint Mobility
ALT	-	Alanine Aminotransferase	LOPS	-	Loss of Protective Sensation
API	-	Association of Physicians of India	MRA	-	Magnetic Resonance Angiography
AST	-	Aspartate Aminotransferase	MRI	-	Magnetic Resonance Imaging
BK	-	Below Knee	MRSA	-	Methicillin Resistant *Staphylococcus aureus*
BP	-	Blood Pressure	MT	-	Metatarsal
CT	-	Computerized Tomography	MTP	-	Metatarsophalangeal
CTA	-	Computed Tomographic Angiography	Na^+	-	Sodium
DM	-	Diabetes Mellitus	NEG	-	Nonenzymatic Glycosylation
DSA	-	Digital Subtraction Angiography	NLD	-	Necrobiosis Lipoidica Diabeticorum
EVA	-	Ethyl-Vinyl-Acetale	PDGF	-	Platelet-Derived Growth Factors
ECG	-	Electrocardiogram	PET	-	Positron Emission Tomography
EGF	-	Epidermal Growth Factor	PTA	-	Percutaneous Transluminal Angioplasty
ESR	-	Erythrocyte Sedimentation Rate	PTFE	-	Polytetrafluoroethylene
FGF	-	Fibroblast Growth Factor	PVD	-	Peripheral Vascular Disease
GCSF	-	Granulocyte Colony-Stimulating Factor	RSSDI	-	Research Society for Study of Diabetes in India
Hb	-	Hemoglobin	SFA	-	Superficial Femoral Artery
HbA_1c	-	Hemoglobin A_1c	TCC	-	Total Contact Cast
HBO	-	Hyperbaric Oxygen Therapy	$TcPo_2$	-	Transcutaneous Pressure of Oxygen Tension
IDF	-	International Diabetes Federation	TLC	-	Total Leucocyte Count
IGF	-	Insulin like Growth Factor	TSP	-	Toe Systolic Pressure
IP	-	Interphalangeal	VCD	-	Video Compact Disc
IVUS	-	Intravascular Ultrasound	VPT	-	Vibration Perception Threshold
K^+	-	Potassium	WHO	-	World Health Organization
KM	-	Kilometer			

Index

READER SUGGESTIONS SHEET

Please help us to improve the quality of our publications by completing and returning this sheet to us.

Title/Author: DIABETIC FOOT: A Clinical Atlas *by Sharad Pendsey*

Your name and address:

Phone and Fax:

e-mail address:

How did you hear about this book? [please tick appropriate box (es)]

☐ Direct mail from publisher   ☐ Conference   ☐ Bookshop

☐ Book review   ☐ Lecturer recommendation   ☐ Friends

☐ Other (please specify)   ☐ Website

Type of purchase: ☐ Direct purchase   ☐ Bookshop   ☐ Friends

Do you have any brief comments on the book?

Please return this sheet to the name and address given below.

JAYPEE BROTHERS
MEDICAL PUBLISHERS (P) LTD
EMCA House, 23/23B Ansari Road, Daryaganj
New Delhi 110 002, India